❧ BODY LANGUAGE ❧

⤚ BODY LANGUAGE ⤙

FIRST OF ALL DO NO HARM

BY

CONSTANCE STUDER

Purdue University Press
West Lafayette, Indiana

Library of Congress Cataloging-in-Publication Data

Studer, Constance.
 Body language : first of all do no harm / Constance Studer.
   p. cm.
 Includes bibliographical references.
 ISBN 978-1-55753-516-0
 1. Studer, Constance. 2. Nurses--United States--Biography. 3.
Convalescence--Psychological aspects. I. Title.
 CT275.S8946A3 2009
 362.16092--dc22
 [B]
                              2009005169

Contents

Acknowledgments

Grateful acknowledgment is given to the editors of the following journals in which these essays first appeared: Earlier versions of "Are You Okay? Yes, I'm Okay" and "Taming the Wolf" appeared in the *American Journal of Nursing,* Diana Masson, Chief Editor, and *Kaleidoscope,* Darshan Perusek, Editor. "Holy Socks" appeared in *Sanskrit,* Michael Kerr, Editor, and in *North Dakota Quarterly,* Robert W. Lewis, Editor. "Solo" appeared in *Mochila Review,* William Church, Editor. "Learning the Language" appeared in *Red Wheelbarrow,* Randolph Splitter, Editor. "Are You Okay? Yes, I'm Okay" appeared in *SLAB: Sound and Literary Art Book,* Autumn Moss and Francine Maitland, Editors. "Inscape" appeared in *South Dakota Review,* Brian Bedard, Editor.

My friends and family have offered loving support in various ways. Some of them have read earlier versions of these essays and given me their comments, for which I am grateful. However, the most valuable support was their belief in me, that I could finish this book. There are so many ways in which my friends have sustained me: a conversation over lunch or on the phone, having dinner after a movie, caring enough to critique my work, or appearing at my bedside during one of my hospitalizations. These are the friends whom I wish to thank: Ruth Taylor, Marcia Lattanzi-Licht, Morgan Songi, Louise Cook, Meri Wilett, Jerrie Ann Hogsett, Ida Peterson, Mary Lou Smith, Linda Hogan, Bobbie Dougherty, Deborah Viles, Connie Oehring, Judith Lavinsky, Susan Boucher, Rebecca Dickson, Sally Green, and Joan Dawson. I will be eternally grateful to Dr. William Shiovitz, Dr. Daniel Hamilos, and Dr. Rajko Medenica for their superb medical care. I thank Cortney Davis and Judy Schaefer, Editors, for including my work in the anthologies, *Intensive Care: More Poetry and Prose by Nurses* (University of Iowa Press, 2003), and *The Poetry of Nursing: Poems and Commentaries of Leading Nurse-Poets,* Judy Schaefer, Editor (The Kent State University Press, 2006).

I am grateful for the loving support of my family: my son, Christopher, my sisters Patricia Hennes, Kathryn Browne, Jeanne Hager, Barbara Mucci and my brother, Charles Browne. And most of all, I dedicate this book to my beloved parents, the Reverend Lucien Adams, Evelyn Adams Browne, and to my stepfather, Dr. Kenneth Browne.

Introduction

This book grew out of my desire to eulogize my father, Reverend Lucien Adams, a Methodist minister who was confined in Toledo State Hospital, Toledo, Ohio, in 1947. I did not attend his funeral in 1963, because it took me a long time to admit even to myself, let alone to the world at large, that my father had vanished from my life because he was diagnosed as a paranoid schizophrenic and was given a prefrontal lobotomy. As this book has evolved through many revisions, I realized that my family's story was part of a larger story about how the medical profession's philosophy "First of all do no harm" can be forgotten or, even more egregiously, be ignored when financial incentives are at stake. If a member of the medical community dares stray from a medical practice deemed "Standard of Care," such as lobotomy in the 1940s or the universal immunization policy in place today, he can find himself ostracized by his peers or perhaps even out of a job.

It was my stepfather, Dr. Kenneth Browne, a family practitioner in rural Ohio, who showed me, by his example, what being a doctor meant: the hardship, the long hours, the commitment required to try to heal the human beings entrusted to his care. All the years I worked as a registered nurse in Intensive Care-Coronary Care and as a hospital supervisor, I considered myself a compassionate nurse. But it was only after becoming a patient myself that I truly understood what patients endure.

An internal medicine physician can perform miracles by prescribing the correct medication that will relieve chest pain or lower blood pressure. Surgeons' skillful hands can remove a blood clot from a patient's brain or reattach a severed finger. However, physicians have a more difficult time dealing with those who live year after year with chronic illnesses. My doctors have saved my life more than once when I was engulfed by yet another medical crisis, but they cannot heal my body. I have been aware of how frustrating this is for them, so difficult to acknowledge or to discuss.

I was working as a registered nurse in Intensive Care-Coronary Care when I was accepted into the Master of Arts program in creative writing at the University of Colorado. It was while I was in graduate school that I came across this observation by Carl Jung: "… Every personality has a story. Derangement happens when the story is denied. To heal, the patient had to rediscover his story."

When my fellow nurses learned that I was taking writing workshops and graduate classes, a curious thing happened. All at once, I was perceived as not being as serious about nursing as I had been before. The thought of changing careers was the furthest thing from my mind. Since no one asked what writing meant to me, I never was given the chance to explain that writing is a way of life as well as a vocation, a process, a journey more than a destination. Writing is a life-sustaining habit, like exercise or eating three meals a day. Writing is a mingling of sweet and sour, yin and yang, terror and tingle. A legal high when a sentence works or a poem tells me what it wants to say, writing is that trancelike state where distractions disappear and endorphins are released, those natural opiates flooding the senses.

Writing and nursing go together like a long marriage where each partner takes turns crying and consoling, arguing and reconciling. The marriage lasts because both partners know they've been heard and understood and accepted in spite of all their imperfections. As a nurse and a writer, I believe that telling a story and listening to another person's story is what sacred means.

Various readers of my book have commented on its combination of poetic as well as narrative style. It was more an intuitive process than a rational decision that convinced me that this would be the best way to present my family's story—my father's lobotomy, my mother's slow decline into Parkinson's disease, and my own experience with systemic lupus—as well as other people's experiences with the darker side of medicine.

Today, most graduating medical students still swear to uphold some form of the oath written by Hippocrates, the father of medicine in the fourth century B.C. This oath delineates the ethical principles by which physicians treat their patients: to treat the sick to the best of the physician's ability; to preserve the patient's privacy; to teach the secrets of medicine to the next generation; to practice and prescribe to the best of the physician's ability for the good of his patients; and most importantly, to never do deliberate harm to a patient for anyone else's interest.

Body Language is a plea to the medical community to demand the release of clinical studies, as documented in Robert F. Kennedy's article, "Deadly Immunity," showing a link between the ever-increasing number of children suffering from autism and the amount of thimerosal, an ethylmercury preservative, they receive every time they are given an immunization. If we are truly an ethical profession, we will demand that vaccines be proven safe before they are administered to the most vulnerable among us, newborn infants. Every parent should be given the opportunity to make an informed decision before immunizing his or her child. Parents have a right to see what illnesses have been reported to the voluntary VAERS (Vaccine Adverse Effects Reporting System, which began in July 1990). Every parent should be told they have the right to refuse to have their children immunized, for whatever reason that parent deems relevant. Why hasn't funding been allocated to an independent clinical institution to follow-up on the thousands of injuries reported to the VAERS system? How are these people doing two, five, or ten years later? Are they still ill? Are they still alive? No one knows because no one has cared enough to follow up on these cases, including my own.

I have been living with systemic lupus for twenty-three years, and it never ceases to amaze me how quickly new symptoms can appear, yet another challenge to face. But, even though I may not be able to heal my body, I have healed my life: spending the morning writing; sitting on the shore of Grand Lake watching ducks float by as hawks do their call-and-response act high up in the trees; sinking down in a warm tub of water; laughing with good friends over life's latest absurdity; making a positive contribution whenever I can; and seeing my grown son prosper as remarkable, successful young man.

Body language is a foreign language slowly translated, often painfully understood. Just to dance, to be, arms up, legs stretching out is a blessing. Constantly testing, teasing the boundaries with a turn of the head, a touch. Breath follows breath. Nothing else matters.

Chapter One

☞ Holy Socks ☜

I was four when my father went into Toledo State Hospital in 1947 and never came home again to live. I have faint memories of his large hands pushing hair out of my eyes and of watching him preach in front of a small church while an organ played "Amazing Grace." He told my sister and me stories about Holy Socks, who was sometimes funny as Father hopped around like a rabbit twitching his nose, swishing his tail. Sometimes Holy Socks was a scary monster who gobbled up any socks left on the floor. The story was never the same two nights in a row. Sitting on the church steps, the world was all dandelions and bluets, smooth green knolls bristling with lilacs and thistle.

Spirit has many meanings. It can mean breath. And then there's "spirited away," a phrase that can mean someone was abducted or perhaps passed on. But most importantly, spirit means having the courage to persevere. My father, a Methodist minister, preached about the Holy Spirit. My sense of the sacred as a child was connected to memories of my father: accompanying him on pastoral calls and hearing him preach every Sunday. As a preacher's kid, I spent a lot of energy wriggling out from under kisses of maudlin matrons to whom religion was a foundation garment that squeezed out all breath, poked them at every step.

In 1963, I was twenty-one and a third-year student nurse at Toledo Hospital School of Nursing. Part of that training was a three-month psychiatric affiliation at Toledo State Hospital, the institution in which my father had been confined since his lobotomy.

"Would you get this chart for me, please?" I asked, handing the elderly woman a slip of paper.

"Why do you want this chart?" she asked.

"I need to do a nursing care study on this patient," I mumbled, avoiding her eyes. My palms were sweaty. "I'm a student nurse."

As she shuffled off to find the chart, I leaned against the wall and took a deep breath. I had no idea what punishment would befall me if my nursing instructors discovered that I had read an unauthorized chart. I needed to find out why my father had spent more than half of his life in Toledo State Hospital. The loss of my father was a cave of silence: the silence of secrets too painful to tell; the silence of a doctor's orders hidden away on dusty charts, long ago destroyed; the silence of the cultural taboo attached to mental illness; the silence of a life lost in the wilderness of back wards where no one visited; the silence of the medical profession's arrogance at playing god with other people's psyches, cutting brain tissue in order to still an argumentative voice, to make a life conform, to cut a life down to size. The old woman trudged back to the counter with two thick manila folders. "You can't take these out of this room," she said. "Bring them back to me when you're through."

As a Methodist minister, my father knew the Bible preached that he must be silent to hear God's guidance, but when he was silent, he was accused of acting strangely. I had so many questions. Was madness the domain of doctors or theologians? Was it caused by physical pathology or spiritual depravity? Was it a disturbance of body chemistry or the result of cultural influences? Had my father spent so much of his life behind locked doors because he loved God so mightily that his circuits blew, madness as a form of prayer?

Many years later I found a newspaper clipping, brittle with age. The editor of the paper in the small Ohio town where my parents began their ministry had written an article about my parents. "Adam and Eve at Home," was the title. He described watching "Eve," my mother, Evelyn, playing the piano, while "Adam," my father, Lucien, sang a hymn. How interesting that the editor would equate my parents with the world's first lovers, the prototype for all those who came after, authors of that ancient story of sin and sex and sorrow and redemption. "Adam" means "blood," "earth," and "the first gardener." "Eve" means "life" or "living." In the beginning, out of nothing, God's spirit brought light, then divided light from darkness. He created Adam, breathing in life and soul. Adam adored Eve, just as my father adored my mother, flesh of his flesh, bone of his bone. "You'll bear children in pain," God said to Eve. "You'll toil in the fields," God said to Adam. They made choices and were forced to live with the consequences. God placed a spinning sword at the mouth of the garden to keep sinners out. Adam and Eve spent the rest of their lives trying to get back where they started.

My father was a romantic, down on his knees in love with my mother, a believer in the true sweet ache of it. Blood rush. Grand holiday of reason. Cheers from the awakened soul. Love, the only glimpse of heaven any of us will ever get. When my mother walked down the aisle of the Ruggles Methodist Church one warm summer evening, the young interim pastor was besotted. One look at her and Father decided brotherly love wasn't the most important kind. He was tall and so thin that his body weaved in and out as he preached. The oak pulpit glowed under its patina of varnish. A purple linen cloth hung down the front. Above the altar hung a simple oak cross. Angels and apostles danced in the stained glass windows. Father was a transcendental philosopher, a dreamer, a writer who tried to make poetry out of sermons. My only legacy from him was a battered notebook in which he scribbled poems and Bible verses and notes for sermons. *Faith is the door we all must knock on, but not everyone gains admittance. The word "bliss" comes from the same word as "wound."* Bliss, that condition known to infants, psychotics, saints, and lovers.

My family had moved every two or three years. The Bishop of the Ohio Conference had the power to uproot lives for many reasons: maybe parishioners had lodged complaints about a true believer's preaching style, his tendency to forget names, or the slope of his haircut. A good minister was one who accepted his calling to another church without question.

Mother was petite and had hair that shone gold in the sunlight. She always seemed, even when seated, to be moving forward at breakneck speed. After the service, Pat and I climbed into the backseat of the Chevy. Home was Whitehouse, Ohio, a small farming community with perhaps two hundred souls when all the aunts and uncles and cousins were home for the holidays. Even then it was a shrinking town with one grocery store and one faded brick drugstore. Hay fields came right up to the edge of Main Street. Almost all Ohio towns looked the same in the late 1940s: a bronze soldier held his rifle in the town square, one church, one bar, one stoplight, and a drinking fountain in front of the drugstore on the corner.

Driving toward the small white parsonage, ghost words fluttered out the window of the car. My mother asked something about a woman in the church having bruises and what could be done. My father pulled her into the shelter of his arm. The parsonage needed a coat of paint, and inside there was a bookcase full of books, a Philco radio where we heard news about the war still raging, a floor lamp, a threadbare rug, and brown sofa rubbed shiny from years of use.

My parents' most prized possession was a piano that was given to my family by someone in the congregation, an heirloom. My father sang in a deep baritone, and my mother joined him in her strong alto harmony, a smile flashing between them. My mother's brow had a permanent groove of worry because of the meager collection plate. I overheard our neighbor, Fern Barker, refer to my family as being as poor as church mice. I thought all little girls wore hand-me-down clothing from their older sister.

Father took me along on his pastoral calls. Every time we went into the nursing home there was the same odor of Clorox, dead flowers, and urine. We walked past men and women in wheelchairs while a woman in a white dress gave out little cups of pills. Low cries and moans followed us down the hall. Doors stood open leading into darkness. Father opened the door to a room where an old man lay in a crib. He put his hand through the side rail and touched the man's shoulder. The man had no hair or teeth, and his eyes were half open. He tried to speak, but there was no sound.

"Show me where it hurts," my father said. His hand moved to his belly. My father pulled up the sheet. His belly was round and shiny.

"Please," the man whispered.

"I'll see if I can get some help for your pain," he said. My father returned with a nurse. She had a glass tube with a plunger, a piece of rubber tubing, and a bottle on a tray. Gently, my father uncurled the old man's arm while the nurse tied rubber tubing around his thin arm and pushed in the needle.

"We'll stay for a while," my father said to the nurse. She was already out the door, onto the person further down the hall who needed her the most.

"There now, Joe, there now," my father crooned, just like he did when my sister and I fell down and cut our knees. Slowly, the old man's face relaxed into a smile. We sat beside Joe's bed until his breathing became quiet and easy and he slept.

On a gray, freezing day in January of 1946, my parents brought my baby sister, Marguerite, home. Hail beat coldly against the northwest windows. It was when my sister and I helped our mother change the baby's diaper that we learned the truth. There was a large hump on her tiny back. It had a purplish cast to it, like a huge bruise. There was a white gauze bandage on her back. Her forehead looked large. No hair. When Mother put her finger in Marguerite's hand, she didn't grab hold.

"What is that on her back, Mama?" I asked.

"Part of her spinal cord is on the outside, instead of on the inside," Mother said softly as she rubbed baby oil into the hump. She lowered Marguerite into a small basin of water.

"Doesn't it hurt?" Pat asked.

"Hurt? No, I don't think she's in pain. It's up to your Daddy and me to make sure she isn't." Mother had to lay the baby on her side or her stomach. The top of her head bulged and I could see her pulse beat there. The smell of the baby, wet scalp, talcum powder, the sour smell of milk. Mother held Marguerite in her right arm and trickled a small stream of warm water over her head and down the tiny chest, belly, and legs. She allowed me to help with this baptism. Mother murmured and cooed, trying to get Marguerite to fix on her face, but my sister's eyes remained vacant. Mother let me put on her diaper and pajamas.

"Do you want to hold her?" Mother asked.

"Will I hurt her?"

"No, honey. Sit in this rocker." Mother put Marguerite in my lap. Her back felt hard against my chest, like a grapefruit. Her eyes peered out of the pink blanket with a look of astonishment, and then she slept.

Fluid wound through the ridges and valleys of nerve cells in Marguerite's brain, like a vast network of underground rivers, spilling into open spaces called ventricles, forming tiny lakes as it made its way back down her spinal cord. Marguerite's pathway was blocked, resulting in an excess of fluid in the brain's canals. If she didn't have surgery, the pressure of the fluid would cause her head to enlarge and create symptoms such as headaches, seizures, vomiting, and problems with her vision. Spina bifida was a strange affliction that had arisen out of the pitch, the accumulation of thousands of years of genetic evolution that had compressed into the single moment of my sister's conception.

My father was in his study working on the sermon he would deliver the next Sunday. Marguerite was eight months old and lay in her bassinette in the corner of his study. Pat had gone to play at the neighbors' house. Mother had gone to the store. I was in my hideout in the back of the downstairs closet. I lay down in the dark on a nest of coats and old sheets that my mother planned to cut up for diapers.

I swam in the darkness of clothes. Tiny drums of bone swept up from the bottom of this lake. I swam within the belly of the house. Feet were running. Doors slammed. I heard my father's voice yelling and then a high-pitched scream. Something about blue and stillness and breath. Breath-less. No breath. Then my mother was home, and there were many people creaking floorboards, answering the phone, slamming doors. Much later I heard my father and Pat calling my name. I didn't answer. I was afraid. Something had happened, and I knew that nothing would ever be the same again. Finally, the house was quiet, and I floated in my silent lake.

"Connie, come out of there, dear." Fern, our next-door neighbor, filled the closet doorway. "Come on sweetheart." Rubbing my eyes, I crawled out with one of my mother's sweaters around my shoulders and my father's hat on my head.

"Something happened to Marguerite," I said.

"Come sit on my lap. I'll try to explain." Fern was large and made a swishing sound from the rubbing of her thighs as she walked. Buttons never exactly brought the edges of her dress together.

"Dr. Browne was here. Your parents have taken Marguerite to the hospital, but there's nothing anyone can do," she said. "She's gone."

"Gone? Where?" I asked.

"God took Marguerite with Him to heaven." Fern held me in her lap. The only sounds in the house were the creaks of the old rocker against the bare floor.

The bells of Whitehouse Methodist Church called. The evening air was thick with lilacs and honeysuckle and spirea. The darkening sky was alive with darting moths and flickering fireflies as we entered the church. At the front of the church my sister lay in her tiny box. A casket, my mother called it. Pat and I were squeezed between our parents on the front pew. The eaves, long and low, rose like bloody bones.

A minister from the next town conducted Marguerite's funeral. I blocked out the words that were supposed to calm and console. Words hurled up into the wilderness of heaven. Words of the hymns vibrated against my temples. If God could take a little baby, none of us were safe.

"Amazing Grace…how sweet the sound…that saved a wretch like me…" As the minister sang, he made a cage of his hands by touching his fingertips as his right hand balanced against his left. "…I once was lost, but now I'm found…" He tilted forward on his toes and then tilted back on his heels, "…was blind, but now I see."

Tears rolled down cheeks. No sense trying to hide them. My mother wiped away the wetness, but more tears just came in their place. My father bowed his head and held his glasses in his lap. All of us held hands, a lifeline to home. Then there was nothing left except to carry the small casket to the cemetery where moonlit stones lay in rows like teeth with nothing to bite but sky.

The Ohio Methodist Conference was held in a barn-like building with open rafters and a wooden floor. Seats clattered as they tipped up and down. My father was just one in the thousands milling about, anxiously waiting to learn whether or not they would be able to stay in their church one more year. Annual Conference was a social club, a Board of Director's meeting, and judgment day all rolled into one.

There were signs designating the different Ohio districts with some of the fervor but none of the power of a political rally. Steubenville. St. Clairsville. Mansfield. Akron. Cleveland. My family sat in the Toledo district. There were committee reports from the chairman of the Caring Cupboards who helped keep food on the table for thousands of families during difficult economic times and a report from the committee that helped widows who had lost their husbands in the war. While these reports were being read from the platform, a steady stream of ministers walked by the open book at the front of the room just below the platform where the Bishop presided. My father joined the line of ministers milling about and chatting in the aisles before they learned their fate.

"This isn't fair," my father yelled. "I can't move again."

"Reverend Adams, you're disturbing the proceedings," the Bishop said. The room was suddenly quiet.

"You can't move me and my family again," my father shouted.

"You're out of line, Reverend Adams. Please restrain yourself."

My father ran down the aisle and out the door into the street. My mother ran behind him but was caught up in the crowd and couldn't reach him before he vanished through the door.

He sat in his car, and somehow the key didn't fit the ignition. He sat there on the corner of Miller and Lincoln Streets and couldn't remember how to drive, how to get his arms to work, how to turn the key, or how to make his right leg step on the gas. A blue light glowed around the steering wheel. Then the car was running, but the white line kept disappearing as he weaved the car through traffic. He rubbed his eyes, but it didn't help. No way to turn the car off, and so he listened to a fountain of voices spraying. Voices boiling the radiator over, voices propping open the hood. Afternoon shadows scattered in a jagged dance. Bushes moved. Sunlight shattered the windshield into glassy stars.

⇒   ⇐

There are times in life when a family's course is forever altered. The damage only becomes apparent much later. Or perhaps too late to be undone. This was one of those times. My mother paced the floor because my father had not come home. It was late at night when the police station rang. The officer told her that my father was safe with them.

When we arrived at the police station, Father was in a room by himself, sitting at a table looking mortified and frightened. He'd lost his glasses and his suit jacket.

"Lucien, we're taking you home," my mother said.

"We need to have him evaluated," the officer said. "We found him sitting in his car. He said he couldn't drive anymore because a voice told him he'd die if he put his hands on the steering wheel. He thinks he killed his daughter."

"Our baby died of a genetic disease. It was no one's fault." She took her husband's hands in hers trying to bring warmth to the ice she felt.

"The psychiatrist will be here later tonight," the officer replied. "Lucien needs to stay here until he sees him."

The doctor who evaluated my father found him oriented to time and place and person, but in his opinion, he was subject to mood swings and limited insight and judgment. My father admitted to hearing God's voice. Based on this information, the doctor diagnosed my father as paranoid schizophrenic and thought he was a danger to himself.

My mother signed the consent form, and on the line asking the reason for my father's admission to Toledo State Hospital, my mother wrote, "Lucien needs rest." She visited the love of her life in a hospital with Goliath structure, a place of parallel trees and concrete buildings that had not aged well. Some delusional architect had tried to enhance the landscape by adding a few turrets and Corinthian columns, but it hadn't helped. The hospital was a squat mess with barred and screened windows. High-pitched voices and cries came from somewhere deep inside.

Mother sat in the psychiatrist's office waiting to find out how she could help her husband. On the wall was the etching of Herr Freud. Sigmund the Conqueror. Monarch over the unconscious, explainer of impulses, unleasher of Ego, master of Id. The doctor told her that my father needed electroshock therapy, and she agreed because she thought that would bring my father home.

Father was wheeled in on a gurney, and his arms were tied to iron railings. They put a wedge under his back and globs of paste were put on both temples. A rubber bridge was inserted between his teeth. The doctor turned a dial on a brown box. Assistants kept his mouth tightly closed around the rubber gag. Someone pressed down on his shoulders as he fishtailed and contorted and convulsed. It was only after the lightning went through his head that the pain in his chest began. His breath came hard. He felt faint and sweaty. Pain shot through his chest upwards to his throat. The pain grew worse. Crushing. He was losing power, a terrifying seepage of strength.

"Maybe it's better this way. Won't have to think about Marguerite anymore, her tiny body a ripple of ribs and belly, her little bones threatening to poke through her skin. Her head almost too heavy to hold."

Suddenly, there was noise, lights, and commotion. Someone gave him nasal oxygen and took his pulse and blood pressure. Abruptly, he was a body pathology instead of a brain pathology, and he smiled at the irony.

"How do you feel?" someone asked.

The elephant sitting on his chest was slowly being replaced by a wolf—a sharp bite but not as much weight.

"Lucien?" the doctor said. "Are you okay?"

"What happened?" he asked.

"I think you had a heart attack," the doctor replied. "I'm putting you in the infirmary overnight."

"Tell Evelyn," my father whispered. If he died without telling her, she'd never forgive him. He laughed to himself, because this was indeed the logic of a deranged mind. The nurse who helped him into a clean hospital gown looked down at her patient's face and wondered why he was smiling.

Father's childhood case of rheumatic fever had weakened his heart. Because he could not tolerate electroshock treatments, the doctor recommended a prefrontal lobotomy. The hospital was full of strange noises at night—hooting owls, howling wolves, and screaming pumas. The night before his surgery, an aide appeared at my father's bedside to prepare him for the surgery scheduled in the morning. The aide told my father to lie on his left side, knees up to his chest, as Paulo was busy behind him with a small pail and rubber tubing.

"Will I be asleep?" my father asked.

"No. The doctor will give you an injection to deaden the skin, but he needs to have you awake so that you can tell him where he is while he's working on your brain. You sort of give him directions," the aide said with a laugh. The fluid was all in. My father leaped toward the commode in the corner of the ward.

"I've changed my mind," he said. "I want to talk to my wife. Can I call her?" he yelled from the commode.

"It's too late to change your mind," the aide said. "Your wife signed the consent. It says on your chart that you're a paranoid schizophrenic. No one's going to listen to your mind. Hey, man, you're a patient in a mental hospital. You're here because your mind is sick."

"Can't I leave if I want to?" he asked.

"In your dreams," the aide replied. "There are only two ways you'll ever get out of this hospital, either in a box or if you have this surgery tomorrow."

Promptly at six a.m., the aide appeared again, this time with shears. A loud swish of scissors and my father's hair sifted down to grey linoleum. There was no turning back. He didn't protest again. Events were moving too fast. "No jewelry," the aide said, so my father took off his wedding ring.

The aide helped him onto the gurney and angled it down the hall. The small room had no spotlights, no banks of sterile instruments. He felt someone put cold liquid on his scalp. First his right arm, then his left arm was tied down.

"The Lord is my shepherd; I shall not want. He maketh me to lie down in green pastures: he leadeth me beside still waters. He restoreth my soul…"

He felt the pinprick of a needle, one, two, three, four times.

"…He leadeth me in the path of righteousness for His Names' sake…"

There was chilling pain as the needle went in, then his head was numb. Behind him he heard a rattling of instruments and suction ready as the doctor made an incision through layers of skin above the frontal lobes of his brain. The doctor sectioned off the left upper quadrant of my father's skull.

"You'll hear a loud noise. You'll feel some pressure, but no pain," the doctor said. My father heard a loud burring noise as the doctor made holes in the left side of my father's skull.

"…Yea, though I walk through the shadow of death, I will fear no evil: for thou art with me…"

The sound of a saw.

"I'm feeling pain," he said. "In the back of my forehead. Doctor, are you there?"

"Of course I'm here," the doctor said. "Where else would I be?" The doctor pulled the plunger on the leucotome, retracting the looped wire into the cannula.

"…Thy rod and thy staff they comfort me…"

He placed the blunt end of the shaft into the hole on the left side of my father's skull two inches below the cortex into the white fibers that connect the frontal lobe to the rest of his brain.

"…Thou preparedest a table before me in the presence of my enemies: thou annointest my head with oil…"

The doctor pressed the plunger on the leucotome and the loop opened. He rotated the device and a core of white brain tissue was severed.

"*…My cup runneth over. Surely goodness and mercy shall follow me all the days of my life.*"

"We're about one-fourth of the way done, Lucien," the doctor said. "Now I'd like you to repeat the Lord's Prayer for me. It's something you know very well, right, you being a minister and all?"

"Our Father who art in heaven…" my father said.

"That's good. Keep going." The doctor withdrew the leucotome to a depth of one and a half inches, depressed the plunger, and removed a core.

"Hallowed be Thy name…"

"Do you know who I am, Lucien?"

"Yes," my father replied. "You're my doctor."

"Are you going to recover and be able to go home?" the doctor asked.

"I want to. If only the pain in my head on the right side would go away." He retched but nothing came up. Someone turned his head to the left.

"Keep saying the Lord's Prayer."

"It's hard to remember," my father said. "Thy kingdom come…I can't remember how it goes."

The third quadrant was severed. My father felt someone checking his blood pressure.

"Where are you?" the doctor asked.

"I've been telephoning from the corner drugstore, but I lost my dime in the machine," my father replied.

"Who were you calling?" the doctor continued.

"Anyone who'll listen, but I'm having trouble getting through," my father said.

"Are you worried?" the doctor asked.

"No," my father replied.

Another core was made an inch below the cortex. The doctor retracted the loop and removed the instrument from my father's brain. Four cores had been cut. My father felt the cloth being removed and his blood pressure being taken and felt pressure as the doctor closed the protective layer over the brain and then the skin.

"How do you feel?" the doctor asked.

"Okay," my father replied. "Just a nervous trembling, like a chill." He felt his arms being released from their bindings and someone putting a bandage on the top of his head. He vomited twice in the room they took him to after the surgery. The head of his bed was elevated, his knees raised. He felt someone take his blood pressure and feel his wrist for his pulse.

Hours later the doctor appeared by his bedside. "How do you feel?" he asked.

"Much better."

"Do you have any of your old fears?"

"No."

"Do you remember being upset when you came here?"

"I was upset, wasn't I? It's not important now."

"What was going through your mind during the surgery?"

"A knife."

"You don't remember how upset you were about the death of your daughter when you came here?"

"Do I have a daughter?"

"Two. Pat and Connie. But the one I'm talking about is Marguerite. Your baby who died."

My father rubbed his eyes with his hand as if it was a magic slate and his memory would return. He looked down at his hands but didn't realize that his wedding ring was missing. He didn't remember to ask anyone to give it back.

⇝   ⇜

After his surgery, my father came home for one visit. A photograph taken during this time showed my family standing in front of a lilac bush in the front yard of the farmhouse that my mother had rented. My mother looked thin. Father was frowning into the sun, his left hand resting on my mother's shoulder like a claim. There was a confusion of shadows, perhaps flowers, between them. My sister, Pat, and I stood in front of our parents. No one was smiling.

Mother proudly showed him her large garden: rows of broad beans, lettuce heads, clumps of carrots, but my father cowered as he entered our new home, as if he no longer knew how his body fit into the universe. His eyes were lowered. The brown couch was in the bay window. The piano that my father loved so much stood in the living room. The only drapes that my family had ever owned covered these windows, too. My mother was always an expert in making do. It was during that weekend that my mother learned that the "regressed behavior" the doctor talked about meant that my father wet his pants and banged his spoon on the table when he ate. While my mother was making dinner, Father wandered away. After an hour of looking, Mother called the police.

"Do you have a picture of him, Mrs. Adams?" the officer asked.

"Yes." Mother raced upstairs to get the photo that was taken of Father when he graduated from theological seminary. He was smiling, proudly holding out his diploma in his right hand, his wavy brown hair shining. His eyes glowed with joy and intelligence. He stood tall and proud.

"This is how he looked before he got sick, before he had the surgery," Mother said.

"What kind of surgery was it?" the officer asked as he scribbled notes.

"Lobotomy—brain surgery," she replied. "The doctor told me that was the only way that Lucien would ever get out of the hospital. I've always only wanted what was best for him."

"Does he have scars, any unusual features that would set him apart?" the officer asked.

"He has a large scar on his forehead and head, but it's almost covered over with hair now," she said. "What hair he has left has turned grey in less than a year. He has trouble concentrating—no attention span. He walks with a stoop as if he's afraid he'll lose his balance." Mother started to cry.

The officers rose from the table, shifted from one foot to the other. "May we take this photo with us?"

Mother wiped her eyes. "Of course."

"Don't worry, Mrs. Adams. We'll find your husband."

"You'll call me as soon as you know anything?"

"Yes." And they were gone.

They found my father standing on a bridge that spanned the Maumee River, more than five miles away from our home. He was huddled by the railing, holding onto it for dear life.

The police car pulled alongside. "Are you Lucien Adams?"

"I can't get over the bridge."

The policemen got out of the car, photo in hand, and compared the picture to his face. They carried him to the police car. Father heard the silence taking shape, weeds starting to split concrete, a flock of geese receding. He lay down on the back seat and covered his face with his hands. He was on his way back to the concrete building, to his bed next to Lorenzo and Joshua, his home. Now maybe he'd be able to sleep.

My father no longer owned his own body, and my mother, out of necessity, gave up all claim. The State of Ohio that had given him shelter in his hour of need now was my father's guardian and had the power to keep him or let him go. Now he was a mental patient who had lost all power to make decisions about his own treatment. My father had read about the prophets in the Bible who went mad on mountaintops, had ecstatic fits alone in the desert, like John the Baptist, Joan of Arc, and St. Francis of Assisi. These people were labeled as "crazy" by those who knew them.

I still carry with me the memory of my father preaching in that small white church and reading from the Holy Scriptures. "If thou wilt diligently hearken in his sight…and keep his statutes, I will put none of these diseases on thee, which I have brought upon the Egyptians: for I am the Lord that healeth thee." And again from the Book of Deuteronomy: "I kill and make alive; I wound and I heal."

When I read his chart, I finally realized why I'd lost my father. I realized that "lobotomy" meant cutting his skull open so that brain tissue could be scooped out, erasing his memory, his conscience, his ability to write sermons, and his ability to tell Pat and me the story of Holy Socks.

Chapter Two
⇒ Light Still Arriving ⇐

It was late at night when my mother aimed the car up the dirt drive of her parents' farm. The Motter homestead was situated between low hills. The house was brick and had stood for over a century. It was the same tumble-down farmhouse where my mother and her two brothers and sister were born. Nothing had changed over the years, except that now there was no paint on the porch, no rosebushes, and no lawn. Grass had been swallowed up as the cornfield crept closer.

"You girls are going to stay with Grandma and Grandpa Motter while I get us moved and find a job," Mother said. Since it was clear that my father would not be able to return to his job as a Methodist minister, my mother had been informed by the Bishop that we would have to move out of the parsonage.

I woke up the next morning beside my sister in a large bed. The floor creaked as I placed bare feet on the wood and used the slop jar. My grandmother was making bread in the kitchen. Open shelves were filled with mason jars of corn and barley. Apricots and peaches and grapes hung by frayed ropes from an open beam. Ears of corn were displayed on the walls like trophies. Grandfather's curses at the horses floated through the door. Skillfully, Grandma placed a mound of dough back in the crock under a moist towel to rise. She wore her white hair in a thick braid coiled like a crown on the top of her head.

If anyone deserved the epitaph "She Kept Busy" on her tombstone, it was Grandma Motter. She pronounced anyone who did not can beans and tomatoes from their gardens as profligates. Shame on them. Canning was a symbol of frugality and virtuous living. There was nothing she enjoyed more than going to the dirt cellar in the dead of winter and pulling one of her jars of stewed tomatoes from the shelf, opening it, and releasing the sunshine inside. Her shelves were arranged by color: deep reds and purples here, pale yellows and greens there.

Summer meant fresh fruit and lots of it—peaches, apricots, and cherries. Grandmother pinched, poked, and sniffed for quality in tomatoes and melons and peaches. From early summer to late fall, the earthen cellar floor was laden with bushel baskets of freshly picked produce and all the paraphernalia for making jams, jellies, and pickles. Sugar, vinegar, paraffin, and spices were spread out on the worktable. My grandmother was Queen of the Fruit

Cellar. She taught Pat and me how to wash jars and peel peaches, but only the Queen arranged peach halves in the jars—and she did so with the eye of an artist.

It was August, ninety degrees in the shade, and felt like one hundred percent humidity in the kitchen when Grandmother decided to put tomatoes up for winter. She sterilized jars, scalded them, and placed the sealed jars in the pressure cooker. Now it was 120 degrees in the kitchen. She cooked the tomatoes, ladled them into jars, and wiped the rims clean. After sealing the jars with paraffin, she screwed on the Kerr lids and tapped the lids with the edge of a knife, the way a musician might strike his tuning fork, listening for the ring that meant they had sealed. She taught my sister and me how to test for hollowness, the sign that the cans were too tightly packed to keep the contents edible, and how to listen for the ring of authenticity. Shiny jars stored in the dark earth cellar were love made visible.

The three months my sister and I spent with our grandparents were full of picking wild raspberries—"fairy hats," Grandma called them. Sundays found us sitting in the pew of the Baptist Church, Grandfather always too busy to join us. The pastor boomed about eternal hellfire and salvation in his throaty pulpit voice. He had the habit of dividing one-syllable words into two: "Sa-ved. Lo-st."

"Praise the Lord," Grandmother cried with her arms open at appropriate intervals through the invocation, the sermon, and the offering. I looked where she was pointing, hoping to see a little slice of heaven between the rough-hewn beams, but all I could see were cobwebs and dust motes along a strand of sunlight.

One day in late August, Pat and I were sitting on the front porch podding peas. It was so hot that even the bees lurched from one rosebush to the other.

"Can't we go to town and get some sherbet, Grandpa?" I asked.

"Please, Grandpa," my sister said. Grandmother balanced a basket of green beans between her knees. Snipping off each end, then snapping them sharply in the middle, she didn't miss a beat.

"Sherbet? We've got something right here a lot tastier than sherbet. Look at all those cherries," he said. Long branches of the cherry tree bent like bows under their burden. Grandfather loped off the porch toward the tree. "I'll get you something better than sherbet." He grasped a branch with both hands, swung his legs out, and walked his legs up the trunk of the cherry tree. We watched in amazement as he climbed higher, until he was hidden from view.

"Doren, be careful," Grandmother said in the tone of voice she usually used when Pat and I had forgotten to do one of our chores. From high up in the tree, my grandfather crowed as a hailstorm of cherries rained down. Grandmother ran forward, holding out her apron to catch the fruit. Pat and I joined in.

"Look," my grandfather said. He dangled from a branch, knees bent over the branch like a gymnast, arms swaying back and forth, his beet-red face smiling down like the sun. There was a loud crack and a great falling of leaves and cherries and twigs. Grandfather fell headfirst. Grandmother and my sister and I crept close, afraid of what we might see. When he opened his eyes, we were relieved. He looked up into my face hovering just above his.

"Aren't those cherries good?" he whispered.

"Better than sherbet any day," I said.

At night my grandparents' house seemed to talk to itself, groaning and muttering in the aching accents of parting joints and ancient beams. It squealed in the wind with a high note of protest, as though its weathered bones were being twisted in arthritic sockets. Some nights I had nightmares, always with me trying to find my father and the little sister I would never know. Sometimes I saw him standing on the bank of Lake Erie, his pant legs rolled above his knees, thigh deep in water. Always in my dream, my father said, "Jump. I'll catch you," but when I jumped, he vanished. I sank beneath green water and awoke struggling for air.

Grandfather was a ruddy man clad in neat, patched overalls. He walked like a bear with his back bowed and arms curled in front of him. He had a belly like a cast-iron stove, and his legs were bent, as if his body were too heavy to carry all the weight. He worked seven days a week on his dirt farm. Land was the only wealth that he had, and it was eroding away with each cloudburst. However, his dark eyes glowed as he talked about his vision of what the farm would look like someday. Later I understood that, in reality, he was in danger of losing everything and had been for a long time. Living on a farm meant that things could always be worse. The farm was like an old love that had left Grandfather long ago but that he still fantasized about because he remembered how good things could be.

The place where he looked most content was in his Victory Garden. He kneeled, picking potatoes and turnips and radishes. The earth swallowed his hands. One sultry day in August, I was helping him dig potatoes. The sky was the color of a tarnished spoon.

"Don't you ever get tired of all this hoeing and the dirt always under your fingernails?" I asked.

"What else would I do?" he replied. "I'd miss the corn and the soybeans. And the grain elevators—skyscrapers of the prairie. And the rivers when the spring rains come—watching how the herons and egrets splash in swampy fields."

"I'd rather be indoors," I said. A crow swooped low like a banker in wingtips about to foreclose.

"I like being my own boss even if it means getting up at five to milk cows," he said. "Detasseling corn. Baling hay. No doubt about it, farming is a hell of a lot of work."

"Don't let Grandma hear you say that."

"What?"

"Hell."

"It's just an expression."

"Not to Grandma."

"You won't tell on me, will you, Connie? You wouldn't do that to your old Grandpa?" He removed his straw hat and wiped his dripping forehead with a red bandana.

"You know I won't." I assured him. We had almost finished the last row when big clouds rolled in. "It's going to rain," I said. I hopped from one foot to the other, barely concealing my delight that I could stop digging potatoes. Large drops of rain started falling, and I danced under them, my face lifted, welcoming its wet kiss. Sweet rain. Blessed rain. "We need to go in now," I said. Grandfather stayed on his knees over the potato row.

"I'm going in," I said

"So go ahead, scaredy-cat. Afraid of a little rain."

There was a brilliant flash and a loud crack. I was halfway to the farmhouse when the first zigzag of lightning hit. One, two, three, and then a great clap of thunder and afterwards perfect silence. Day became dusk within minutes. Just as I turned to call to Grandfather, another spear of lightning sliced the dark sky. Suddenly, my grandfather became a fluorescent silhouette against the horizon. His arms stood straight out from his body, his face turned to heaven. A light ran through his head and chest and legs, nailing him to Earth. There was the smell of burning flesh.

My grandmother and sister ran across the open field as rain came down in curtains. I ran back too, and by the time we reached Grandfather, he was lying stretched out, face down.

"Is he dead, Grandma?" my sister asked.

"Dear Lord save us. He's still breathing," Grandmother said. With a great lugging and pulling, we turned Grandfather onto his back. His face was the color of slate, but his chest heaved up and down.

"I can't see," Grandfather said.

"Sweet Jesus. Saints preserve us," Grandmother said. "Just like Saul on the road to Damascus, the great light from heaven, the scales on the eyes. Just say you believe, Doren. Just say you believe."

"I ain't that far gone," Grandfather said, as he struggled to sit up. He rubbed his arms. The faint smell of singed flesh lingered in the air.

"Do you think you can walk, Doren?" Grandmother asked.

"I think so, but you'll have to lead me." With Grandmother and my sister on each side and me out in front like a Seeing Eye dog, we managed to get Grandfather back to the farmhouse.

For the next week, Grandfather rested on the couch in the dining room. Grandmother rubbed white ointment into the burns on the palms of his hands and the soles of his feet. It was two whole days before he could see again. He was quieter than usual as he lay on the couch, clutching his cold pipe between yellow teeth.

"The Lord has spared you for a reason," Grandmother told him as she changed the gauze bandages on his hands.

"Don't start with your religion talk," he said. But he let her touch him, let her fetch his pipe and tobacco and cool bandages for his hands. The rest of us fed the chickens, the hogs, and the horses. One night I saw Grandfather standing in the backyard looking up at the moon. His lips were moving, but I couldn't hear what he was saying. He still refused to attend church with Grandmother, but I never heard him swear at the horses again.

⌒ ⌒

My mother grew up during the Depression. Grandfather often made his four children stay home from school to work in the fields. The farm barely eked out a living. Often at dusk, my mother was still standing in the middle of an acre of potatoes. "No supper until that field is clean," her father had told her. "I don't want to see one weed." She often didn't finish her work until well after dark and arrived home long after everyone else had eaten.

"That's why I wanted to get off the farm so badly," Mother said. "I hate dirt under my fingernails." She learned how to barter a dozen eggs with the grocer for a banana or piece of bread or orange. Each day he seemed to take longer before making his decision. He turned each egg, slowly checking for flaws. The grocer drove a hard bargain, and many days my mother had no lunch at school.

That summer when I was four, I watched my grandmother stir a large pan of grey liquid on the kerosene stove that would become brown soap. She added lye and pig lard to make it the right consistency. First came the melting, the cooking, the pouring, and finally the cutting into bars. She added crushed rose and lilac and aster petals in an attempt to mask the strong smell.

"Did Mama walk to school?" I asked.

"No, there was a horse-drawn wagon," she replied. "Evelyn and Ted and Kathryn waited for it at the end of the driveway. I'll never forget the day when your mother was seven, and Ted got on first and helped Kathryn climb on, but Evelyn was halfway up the step when the horses took off. The wagon door slammed shut in her face, and there she was, balancing on the back step, hanging on with her right hand, and hugging her books and a bag containing eggs for barter for bread or ham with her left. Hanging on for dear life until the driver stopped for kids further up the road." Grandmother finished cutting the brown soap into squares, picked one up, sniffed it, and set it back down on the table with a long sigh.

Grandmother's garden was a stash of color: buttercup, canna, and black-eyed Susans. Dragonflies glinted in the sun. Cumulus clouds floated serenely in the blue sky. Round and round I ran, chasing the chickens until sweat clouded my vision. Hens huddled by the wire fence, clucking their advice on survival. There was the sweet smell of decaying hay as I entered the barn. Dust particles danced on sunbeams angling their way through cracks in the wall, like diamonds on an invisible string. When I looked to the right of the wand of sun, the dust was invisible, but a second later, they were visible again. A miracle, the way soap dissolves in warm water. The way nightmares go away in daylight.

Out in the fields with Grandfather, warm soil felt good between my fingers, against my bare feet. I heard the stirrings of alfalfa and grasshoppers. Twilight always brought its colorful peace, a coppery sheen to the fields, and settled disputes between crows as dusk leaned hard against the old farmhouse and then retired.

Every Saturday night Grandma gave me a bath in a large tin tub in the kitchen. She heated the water in a kettle on the stove, then poured it into the tub, one trip after the other.

"Come here, child," she said, as she knelt on her right knee, testing the water with her fingertip. She helped me out of my jeans and shirt and lifted me into the tub. Brown soap that she had made herself rolled over the washcloth before she applied it to my back. Lying in the bath water, I saw Grandma's white nightgown on the clothesline. Formless and fluorescent, it caught the starlight. The sky was a planetarium without walls, stars free of charge. No wind. Even the barnyard was silent. And then the white cloth ballooned out, lifting its sleeves, as if someone had just put it on. Light was still arriving from that distant source, like the flicker of candles in God's lantern.

During the summer that I was four, I thought any moment I would hear my father's voice telling me to hurry up because the pancakes were ready. He would be waiting by the table when I came down the stairs. Once again, I would hear him read from his Bible about hell and heaven, about Judas and Jesus. I believed a miracle would make everything right. Somewhere across the rolling hills of Ohio, my mother was planting corn and beans. She was hanging our old white curtains in new windows. Far away, my father followed behind the Keeper of the Keys, King of the Bathroom Privilege, Doler Out of Cigarette Bounty.

But my grandmother was there, touching me with her pale fingers as faithful as stars, applying strong soap to every crease and fold of my small body, just as she had to my mother's body, hands bestowing their legacy of strength, gentleness, and endurance.

Chapter Three

⌒ SOLO ⌒

Because we had to be out the door by seven thirty each morning, my mother hung our wet laundry out on the clothesline before five. She said she knew how the day would go by whether robins kissed and cooed as she stepped into the backyard. A good laundry day was a billowing breeze from the north that bent sheets forward and back, as if they'd just been ironed. She propped up the sagging line of jeans, blouses, and flannel nightgowns with a forked pole. Hanging up wet clothes promised new beginnings. Gathering in clean clothes, fragrant with Ohio sun, was healing.

My mother entered the solitary existence of being a single parent in the early 1950s when it was uncommon. She wrestled with a budget, learned how to change a flat tire, and how to file income taxes. Her boss often made her work overtime. Mother didn't get invited to dinner because wives were wary, husbands nervous. Although we moved to a town less than thirty miles from Whitehouse, her former friends never called. She had lost her identity as a minister's wife and struggled to find a new fit.

"There's nothing more we can do for Lucien," the doctors told her a few months after my father's lobotomy, and so she divorced him. Mother was in survival mode. When she wasn't typing and taking shorthand for her boss in Toledo, she was working in the quarter of an acre garden she had planted. There were tomatoes and green peppers and potatoes. Behind them were long-nurtured asparagus, raspberry, and strawberry beds. An edible landscape.

"This garden is all that stands between us and hunger next winter," my mother said.

Early May rain washed away rows of seeds. Mother planted again. By late June, she stood on the back porch of the farmhouse and looked with pride at the results of her hard work. Corn stalks leaned full ears low, as if they were straining to hear the Earth's secrets. Tomatoes acquired their crimson blush.

Every morning she rose before dawn, got Pat off to school, and took me to a babysitter in town. She bundled me up in pajamas and blankets so that I could go back to sleep, but I rarely did. "Be a good girl. See you tonight, honey," she said. Once her day of typing and dictation began, my mother had no time to worry about her daughters. Over the nine years that she was a single parent, my mother emerged from the typing pool to become the private secretary of the CEO of the firm. After eight or nine hours at the office, Mother returned home to begin her other ten-hour shift: picking up the house, preparing supper, checking my sister's homework, reading us a story, and tucking us into bed.

Each day brought new discoveries: the haymow with a rope that I could swing across from one side to the other, wagons filled with wheat, and bales of hay stacked to the ceiling connected by spiders' lace. A man plowed the fields, his legs too short for his large body. He waddled as he walked behind his Percherons that pulled a plow.

"Come on Olga, come on Herman," he called to the horses. "Move a little faster there."

I saw the farmer who plowed the fields around our house a lot that first summer, always from a distance through green catalpa leaves. One August day he rounded the corner of the barn just as I settled down on Olga's ample back.

"Ha! Caught you," he said. "What are you doing?"

"I just wanted to see what it felt like to sit on a horse," I said, bracing my muscles for a quick escape.

"What does it feel like?" he asked.

"Like straddling the whole world," I whispered.

"Yes," he said. Hoe in hand, Mr. Fondessey waddled back through the open door and disappeared around the corner.

Ohio winters were so cold that eyelashes froze together without warning. A cup of boiling water tossed into the air turned into a puff of snow before it hit the ground. At the Toledo Zoo, polar bears' feet froze and left bloody footprints in the snow. A banana froze hard enough to pound nails as the temperature plunged to thirty below zero. The same snow that fell in January was usually still on the ground until Easter.

The winter I was in third grade broke new records for northern Ohio. Ten below zero. Snow had been falling all day. The chills started between arithmetic and English, and I could no longer hide my shaking shoulders. Mrs. Nelson bundled me up with vague mumblings under her breath, "Some parents have no sense." Wrapped tightly in long underwear and leggings, I felt myself being carried on the bus down the gravel road towards home. There was no motor sound, only the snow's icy fingernails scraping glass.

The driver helped me off the bus and then shut the door and headed back to town. Left standing in the yard, I stumbled toward the porch where my stiff fingers found the house key in the potted plant. Somehow I couldn't get my fingers to open the door. Icicles hung from the eaves, from poles in clusters, from the elbows of trees, and emerged from eave spouts like muscular arms.

I sat there on the porch crying, my knees drawn up to my chest trying to conserve heat, trying to forget the aching in my arms and legs and back. Mr. Fondessey's leather hat appeared over the railing.

"What is it?" he asked.

"I can't get in the house," I replied. "Mama's at work and my teacher sent me home.

My arms and legs hurt." The key turned obediently in his hand. Gently, he wrapped me in two blankets and set me down on the furnace grate. I heard him go the basement and shovel coal into the furnace and finally warmth floated upwards turning afternoon shadows from blue to orange.

"Mrs. Adams, please?" He said into the phone. "Yes, I'll get her into bed and call Lola to stay with her until you get home." Our neighbor helped me into my pajamas and into bed. Everything was hazy. It was as if I was seeing myself on the wall, only my arms were wrapped tightly in ivory linen. Someone tried to help me stand up. A man held out his hand, but I couldn't reach it because my hands were bound. Figures painted in gold leaf flickered on the wall. Water flowed down my face. My body ached as fever slipped my skin down around my feet and unzipped my spine, threatening to snap me away like wash on my mother's line. Once again I heard church bells tremble in the air.

My temperature was 102 degrees by the time Mother arrived home. She bundled me off to see Dr.Grady, a quiet man with a quarried face and gentle hands, the only doctor in Elmore.

"Her temperature is 103.4," he said. "She has a kidney infection according to my tests. We need to put her in the hospital. She could have long-term problems if we don't treat it aggressively. We need to get the infection under control."

Mother drove me directly to Fremont Hospital. I was admitted to a room with two beds, both empty. I chose the bed by the window.

"Will you stay?" I asked.

"For a bit," she replied. "I'll read to you a while." She read *Black Beauty* until I started to nod off.

"If you need anything, just ring this bell. I'll be back tomorrow evening." She kissed my forehead and was gone. I turned my face away from the door so that I wouldn't have to see her leave. Half-asleep, fever images flooded my mind. The snow had stopped. Ice crystals formed a lacey pattern on the window. I concentrated on trying to find a shape I could recognize: a dolphin, horse, or dog.

I was aware of white forms floating in and out of the room during the night. Early the next morning a nurse breezed in and opened the curtains. She was dressed in a starched white cotton dress and a white cap. "Good, your temperature is almost normal," she said as she removed the thermometer from my mouth. "The antibiotic is working, but we're still not there yet."

She retrieved a metal basin from the bottom shelf of my bedside stand and hummed at the sink as steam rose around her face. The bath ritual began as she scrubbed my body, applied powder and fresh blue pajamas.

"Climb out of bed for a few minutes, dear," she said. "I'll give you fresh linen."

Another nurse entered bearing sheets and quickly the two women ripped off soiled sheets, threw a crisp sheet high over the mattress, then caught the falling edge and tucked it in top and bottom as if they were dancing: three steps to the top of the bed; three steps to the bottom; pull the cloth tightly until it snaps; tuck it in the envelope; draw sheet; top sheet; faded green spread. The women were a duet of efficient movement as they swept soiled linen into the open mouths of pillowcases, wiped off the nightstand, and filled my aluminum decanter with fresh water.

On the sixth day, the nurse awakened me in the middle of the night. A bad accident was coming in, and they needed my bed. She put me on a gurney and parked me in an alcove in the hall. "Ring this bell if you need me," the nurse said as she set the brakes on the gurney. It was a small metal bell, the kind used in hotel lobbies. Voices came out of a black box in the ceiling. Sirens wailed. It was hours before I slept again. The next morning Mother took me home.

"I don't like the way you look," she said, trying to shovel food into my mouth. My pajamas hung in folds because I had lost weight. I didn't even protest staying in bed. She piled comic books on my bed and brought in the radio so that I could listen to "Amos and Andy," "Let's Pretend," and "The Shadow." "*Who knows what evil lurks in the heart of men? The Shadow knows.*"

"Dr. Grady wants you to stay home from school for six months," Mother said.

"Why?" I asked.

"He says it's too dangerous," she replied. "We can't risk you getting another kidney infection caused by streptococcus. I called the school, and they'll send a tutor so that you can stay up with your class." Before Mother left for work each morning, she helped me settle in for my day on the living room couch. She left my medicine on a nearby table and the radio turned on.

Everything took too much energy. A great drowsiness came over me, as though the air was webbed, and I lay trapped within its net. If there was nothing to be done, I was the girl to do it. The hours of convalescence dragged. It was a good day when I could slip into Nancy Drew's healthy body and jump off balconies, catch the bad guy, and forget that I was sick. Books were my teacher, my friend, my inner cave where I was safe.

"Mrs. Rader will check on you at noon and bring you lunch," Mother had told me. Pat left on the school bus. Coal turning over in the furnace below lulled me with its rhythm. I passed time reading the Bobbsey Twins and Cherry Ames. I listened to a soap opera, "Helen Trent," until lunchtime. "*Can a young girl from a mining town in Montana find happiness in the big city?*" By the middle of the day, I was bored and very aware of creaking floorboards and the groan of coal.

It was during those months that I learned the difference between loneliness and solitude, figuring out how to fill the hours when my mother was at work and my sister at school. Loneliness was the snowstorm I had to brave to reach the safety of feeling comfortable being alone with my books and radio music and fleeting sun reflecting off the window. Loneliness was being afraid that every new noise, a car going by outside or a howl from the woods behind the house, meant that I was in danger. Solitude was knowing that whatever occurred during my day alone on the living room couch, I would handle it. Solitude was looking forward to seeing Mrs. Rader's smiling face when she brought me my soup and sandwich at noon. Solitude was seeing the pile of books decrease as I devoured one after another.

Fit, wholesome, hale, robust, hearty, mentally healthy, physically sound. There are many adjectives denoting health, that balance of natural forces, the flow of dark to light. Health is when you are visible as you lie in a hospital bed, and they come when you ring the bell. Healing is having respect for mystery, letting go of mastery, and embracing wonder. I returned to school the following fall.

Christmas was popcorn and cranberry garlands, homemade snowflakes made out of an old lace tablecloth, and paper angels. We had just finished decorating the tree two years after we had moved to our new house when the doorbell rang. We seldom had callers and never on Christmas Eve.

A man and a woman stood on our doorstep. Snow swirled around them. "Evelyn Adams?"

"Yes," she said, opening the door wide.

"We're from the Salvation Army. These presents are for your family. Merry Christmas."

Just as quickly, the two angels were gone. Although we usually opened presents on Christmas morning, Mother said we could open them that night. There was coffee and rice and wheat and sugar and homemade cookies. There were winter coats for my sister and me and a sweater and a check for our mother.

One night, a few months later, we were getting ready for bed. Mother stood in the bathroom in her turquoise bathrobe, brushing her auburn hair, the color of finely pulled taffy. My sister was winding her blonde hair onto metal curlers. I was playing with my collection of plaster horses, pretending they were parading to wild applause.

"Quick, girls," Mother hissed. "Quick now."

Already she was running from the bathroom into the dining room, flicking off lights as she went. The only light left was the ruby glow that rose through the furnace grate. Holding hands, Pat and I ran into our mother's bedroom. The walls were eggshell blue and held a framed picture of "The Last Supper" and there were small blue bottles of Evening in Paris perfume on the dresser. It was only after we were all three in bed, Mother and Pat on the outside and me sandwiched in the middle, that anyone spoke.

"What's wrong?" Pat asked.

"Shh-shh," Mother said. We watched as she leaned over the edge of the bed. At first I couldn't make out what the long, slim object was, until Mother laid it over her left arm like a rifle. I ran my fingers over the surface: wood, smoothly sanded with a gently tapering stem. A baseball bat. My mother kept it under her bed, and I had never suspected.

"There was a man looking in the bathroom window," she whispered. "Be quiet now. The doors and windows are locked. I don't want to risk going to the phone. We'll just stay here together. And if he dares try to get into this house…if he dares…"

She didn't have to finish the sentence. It didn't take much imagination for me to see a skull indented by my mother's strong arm. I wondered if it could be my father, if he could have escaped the hospital, but I didn't want to make my mother feel bad by asking.

"Do you think he's gone?" I asked.

"Yes," she replied. "We're safe. Go to sleep, honey."

Just before dropping off to sleep, I saw Mother return the bat to its resting place under the bed. That night my dreams were filled with white beaches as far as I could see, waves washing everything clean, water rushing in and out. A man rose to the surface just out of reach and then sank below the saltwater frame. Our house was once again still.

⌇ ⌇

Mother parked the car in front of a large concrete building encircled with a metal-spiked fence. My sister and I followed our mother through the bronze doors and down a grey hall that smelled of mildew and bleach.

"How is he today, Henry?" Mother asked.

"You've caught him on a good one," the man said picking up a large set of keys. We followed him down the hall to a small room where my father waited. He stood beside a chair, his lips moving, his eyes on the floor. He started to walk toward us as we entered the room, then sat down slowly on the chair, back hunched, staring in front of him without moving.

"How are you, Lu?" Mother asked, kissing him on the cheek.

"It rained last night," he said in a monotone.

"Did it?"

"I wanted to cross nineteenth street, but I couldn't figure out how to cross the street."

"Where did you want to go?"

"I don't know. No one was here to tell me."

"Give your father a kiss, girls," Mother said motioning us over, but my sister and I stayed where we were. This was not the father who had carried us on his shoulders and told us stories.

"When I see blood when I see blood I'll pass over you," Father shouted as he stood and ran to the far side of the room. He crumpled to the floor hiding his face in his hands.

"Come on, girls, we'd better go. We're upsetting him," Mother said as we motioned to the man with the keys that we were ready to go. We were silent on the drive home. Mother's face was in the shadows, but when we passed a streetlight, I saw that she was crying.

"Why has this happened to Daddy?" Pat asked.

"Your grandmother would probably say that God was putting us to the test," she replied. "Like the Bible says, when Abraham took his son Isaac and put him on a bonfire, willing to offer him as a sacrifice to God. But God didn't let him kill his son. He was only testing his faith."

"Do you believe that?" I asked.

"No," she said. "I don't believe God makes bad things happen to people. He just gives us strength to get through bad things when they do happen. And they happen to everyone sooner or later."

⌇ ⌇

Mental illness may hit one member of a family like a bomb, but shrapnel injures others in the family as well. After his lobotomy, inside my father's brain there were feuding neighbors constantly overstepping their boundaries and actors speaking lines from different plays at the same time. In this new universe in which he found himself, the laws of gravity, economics, justice, biology, government, and even jungle didn't apply. In his mind, my father was driving on the wrong side of the road, convinced only he was right, trying to pass an exam when all the questions were written in hieroglyphics. In his mind, the survival of the human raced depended on whether or not he could keep from blinking his eyes.

Children learn about love by watching their parents. When my father left, that part of my education was interrupted. I learned that love could be dangerous. Love could disappear. No doubt Mother was lonely after the divorce. No one whispered her name in the night. During the months that I slept with her after moving to the farmhouse, I heard her crying into her pillow. Now she was that solitary girl in the Hopper painting, the usherette in a brightly lit but empty theater.

There were many years when my family's social life revolved around Mother and her dates. Pat and I went with her to the dance held every Friday night in the Odd Fellows Lodge in a nearby town. The floor of the barn-like room shone under its waxy film. Card tables and folding chairs lined the walls. Lights were dim. Six men in jeans and flannel shirts swung into a waltz. *"I was waltzing with my darling the night they were playing the beautiful Tennessee waltz."* A tall man with a red shirt and a slow drawl asked my mother to dance. She glided away in the stranger's arms, whirling to a place where I couldn't follow. During those years, there were many mornings when Pat and I awoke to find Hillis sitting at our kitchen table.

"Morning," my mother said, looking relaxed and happy. "What do you girls want for breakfast?"

"Got to go," he said, kissing my mother.

The fringe benefits for daughters of an attractive mother were that we saw Esther Williams swim her way through many romances, saw *The Unsinkable Molly Brown* and *Quo Vadis* and *The Robe* and *Holiday On Ice*. The downside was that I missed my father and didn't understand what had happened to him because Mother rarely talked about the situation. I don't remember Grandmother and Grandfather Adams because Mother never took us to see them. I don't remember my mother ever discussing sex with me except in terms of warnings: be careful in the gym, keep your legs together, be careful of strange men with candy. Virginity, like the cellophane wrapping on a candy bar, was supposed to show my prospective husband that I had been untouched by a human hand. Of course, that also meant that I wouldn't know the difference between a great lover and a novice.

All I knew about love between a man and a woman was what I read in books: love, that glittering gold of emotion, the blood of poem and song. Love was the Old Testament's Jacob taking Rachel's hand in marriage after he had been forced to serve her father for seven years, then seven more. "And they seemed but a few days because of the greatness of his love." Love was a faithful Romeo in the famous balcony scene with his

Juliet. It was love that sent Orpheus, the musician of Greek mythology, into Hades to find his wife, Eurydice. Love sent Sir Lancelot to the rescue of Guinevere. Nightingales sang their lovesick ditties, and so many phrases remind one of romance: love taps, loving cups, love birds, love potions. And those who lost their lovers left secret scratchings on the wall. "*Who gives this woman to this man?*"

The 1950s were a time of sexual bartering: male urges exchanged for female sexual and domestic services. Eisenhower was president. Even my family could afford a television. The Iron Curtain had been torn down between East and West Germany. Medications like Thorazine and Lithium were now being used in mental hospitals to calm fear and anger, but it was too late to help my father. I was eleven the night Mother told my sister and me that we were going to have a visitor the following Sunday.

"Who?" we asked.

"An old friend from Whitehouse," she said. "Dr. Kenneth Browne. He was an elder in your daddy's church. He's the only doctor in town."

A stooped man with spectacles, a pug nose, and receding brown hair arrived promptly at noon. A small blonde girl and red-haired boy clamored out of the car behind him.

"Girls, this is Dr. Browne and his children, Barbara and Charlie." The little girl with tight ringlets clung to one of her father's legs and peeked out. The small boy raced toward my bicycle and picked it up.

"That's mine," I said.

"Bet I can ride it," Charlie said.

"No, you can't, because I won't let you," I replied.

Mother looked pale. She opened her mouth and then closed it tightly. Charlie picked up a handful of sand and threw it in my face. Dr. Browne retrieved his son and Mother took me in the house to wash my face. That was my introduction to my new family.

When Dr. Browne had lost his wife to cancer, Mother sent him a sympathy card, and they started corresponding. Dr. Browne was the doctor who had come to our home the day my baby sister, Marguerite, had died. That was the way a round robin of Sunday picnics and drives by the river and going to Isaly's for ice cream began.

Mother was reading a letter at dinner one night a few months later when her face became deep rose. "He's asked me to marry him," Mother said.

"What?" I asked.

"He wants me to be his wife," she replied.

"You don't want to, do you? I mean you don't know him, do you?" Pat asked, but Mother wasn't listening. She danced around the room, holding the letter to her breast.

On the day of the wedding, one of mother's friends helped her get ready. "Are you sure, Ev?" Dottie asked as she smoothed down Mother's hair.

"As sure as anyone can be before they step out of the belly of a plane wondering whether their parachute will open," she said. "Kenneth is a good man, a good provider."

"I've heard stories about his kids. Charlie threw a lamp out of a window a few weeks ago."

"I'll put a stop to that mighty quick," Mother said. She wore a beige suit, pillbox hat, and white gloves, a proud bride all glide and grace. We four children sat in the front pew as the minister declared us a family: me, eleven years old, in a lavender nylon dress, white gloves, and patent-leather shoes; Pat, a willowy fourteen-year old; Barbara, an eight-year old with gold curls and the innocence of a street urchin with full-tilt cuteness; and Charlie, a wiry six-year old with red hair and a temper to match. Our family doubled in size overnight. I didn't know what to call my new father, and so far I had avoided this problem by not calling him anything.

"Do you take this man to be your lawfully wedded husband?" the minister asked.

"I do," my mother said. A stranger I didn't know put a ring on her hand, gave her a kiss, and led his bride back down the aisle. As for me, I would need to learn the lessons of loneliness and solitude all over again.

Chapter Four

 COMING HOME

Maybe things would have turned out better if all six of us hadn't gone on the honeymoon. "We'll become a real family," my mother said as I watched her brush her hair. It was copper, and when the light hit just right, shot through with gold. "It'll give us a chance to know each other," she continued as she smoothed on her night cream.

"Where are we going?" I asked.

"Letchworth State Park," she replied. "There are trails where we can walk and a lake where you can swim. And we can ride horses, too." Horses were souls to whom I could relate since one of the high points of the nine years we had lived in the farmhouse near Elmore was sitting on Herman's back, one of Mr. Fondessey's Percherons, and riding our neighbor's gelding down the road at a full gallop.

Early in the morning the day after the wedding, there we were wedged into the car, Mother and the father-whom-I-had-not-yet-named, Charlie in the front seat, and Barbara, Pat, and me in the back.

"I want to sit in the middle," Charlie wailed, flinging his small body against the dashboard of the car. "I've got to sit next to you." Mother waited for her new husband to say something, but he was busy studying the map in his lap.

"You're okay where you are, dear," he said.

"No, I wanna sit in the middle," Charlie said as he banged his head against the window. Mother's face was bright red. Pat and I exchanged a look, expecting swift maternal justice, because we knew what would have happened to us if we had tried a stunt like that.

"All right, just this once," my new father said as his small son crawled over my mother's lap to sit between them. With the blind courage (some might call it naiveté) of explorers taking off for a new frontier, we drove the highway north toward Letchworth State Park, a lush, succulent, and peaceful place until my family arrived. My new father had rented two cabins that sat side by side, the plan being to have the newlyweds in one cabin and the four children in the other.

Sunday, and there we were, spit polished and neatly pressed, marching into church together, the Browne family filling one pew. No one in the church heard the sermon because my little brother kept sliding down and lying under the pew. Mother pulled Charlie up and

33

he slid down again, beating his feet against the floor. This time my new father retrieved his son and carried him down the aisle and out the front door. Mother gathered up the rest of us and followed.

Charlie insisted on sleeping with his father, even though Pat and I tried to bribe him with candy and a bedtime story.

"Has he been sleeping with you at home?" my mother asked her new husband.

"I'm afraid so," he said sheepishly. "After Kathryn died, he got in the habit."

"I understand," she said. "Connie slept with me, too, the first couple of months we were on our own."

Three people shared the bed during my mother's honeymoon.

⌐ ⌐

Whitehouse had not changed one iota in the nine years that we had been gone. It was still a place where the mating habits of starlings were a topic of conversation at the local diner. People still grieved the coming of winter because they wouldn't see bare earth until spring. Sun-deprived citizens reassured each other that they would survive March blizzards. The barbershop quartet still performed its tightly ratcheted harmonies at Grange meetings.

Home was a large Victorian brownstone, with a porch cupping the front. My new father was the only doctor in town. On one end of the porch was our home, and the other end was my stepfather's office. Many times, a man with a cut arm or a woman carrying a sick baby rang the bell at the wrong door, and my mother had to tell them that medical help lay at the other end of the porch.

The living room had a walnut open-beam ceiling and a brick fireplace. There was a piano, a dining room with a walnut table and chairs, and a sideboard that contained Haviland China. There were antique walnut lamp tables with marble tops and Tiffany lamps that gave off an amber-green glow. Upstairs there were four bedrooms. Mother and her new husband had one, Charlie had one, Barbara had one, and Pat got the last bedroom.

"Where am I going to sleep?" I asked.

"You can either share with Pat, or we could make this space by the attic stairs into a bedroom for you," my mother said.

"But there's no door," I replied. The space was more an alcove than a room, but it did have a small balcony off to the side.

"We'll get a portable closet and put it by the entrance. That'll give you privacy," she said.

A week later, my stepfather pulled me aside after breakfast. "Let's you and me go to Toledo and get you some new clothes," he said. "You need some before school starts. You're going to be a seventh-grader this year." He waited patiently as I tried on coats and dresses and sweaters. Always a tomboy, for the first time I saw possibilities as I twirled in front of the mirror—maybe if I curled my hair or trimmed my bangs so that people could see my eyes.

Driving home, I looked at my new father's reflection in the twilight. He smoked a cigarette, bent over the steering wheel, a faint smile making permanent wrinkles around his lips and eyes.

"You don't talk much, Connie. Everything okay?" he asked.

"I don't know what to call you."

"What do you want to call me?"

"I've already got one Daddy."

"I know."

"I guess I could call you Dad Browne. Is that okay?"

"That would be fine. I want to adopt you and Pat. What do you think?" His puffs on his cigarette became more rapid.

"I guess that would be okay." My new father wasn't big on talking, but when he did, it was always something important. We drove toward Whitehouse with silence covering us like a warm quilt.

My mother always said that her stepchildren drove her to the Lord. She said it with such vigor that I knew, in her mind, the Lord Himself was chauffeur of the gold limousine. Instead of our new family blending, warring factions emerged. Barbara and Charlie were on a guerilla mission with Mother as their target. She refused to duck or wear camouflage or wave a white flag of surrender. Pat and I didn't know what was happening and so retreated into our own teenage minds, trying to solve new problems: how to make new friends in a new school, how to find our place in a family that we were still getting to know. We were recruits in boot camp, still stunned to find ourselves in a war for which we had never volunteered.

"Fish or cut bait. Wise up about Barb and Charlie. Make them mind what I say," Mother said to Dad Browne over and over. He was a peacemaker in the extreme. Mother tended to see his good nature as weakness. Her purpose in life became "making those kids mind."

Ice skating on the local quarry was the social hub of our small town. I learned to skate in front of bare-boned trees and rocky ledges and bonfire warmth. Hands plunged deep into the pockets of my parka, I skated as fast as I could, frozen air racing past my face. Light from the bonfire was reflected in the ice passing under my skates like an illusion as I skated in circles until my legs trembled and ankles caved.

One evening after skating, I stood in the bathroom with my mother. She combed her hair while I brushed my teeth.

"What would you say if we left here?" Mother asked.

"Leave? What do you mean?" I spit out the toothpaste.

"I don't know if I can do this," she said, turning her back to me.

"This is home. Where would we go?"

My mother left the bathroom in a hurry. The subject never came up again. The following month, my mother and stepfather announced that we would have a new addition to our family.

Mother was a Depression child and never got over being afraid that someone would take her food away, that she would have to sprout potatoes alone in a dank cellar. Even after she married my stepfather, she carried her purse with her from room to room, afraid to let it out of her sight.

When I was fourteen, Mother stopped going to the Methodist Church with the rest of the family, the same church where my father had been pastor so many years before, the church where my stepfather was a leader. She joined the Christian and Missionary Alliance Church in Toledo.

"I've been born again," Mother announced one night at dinner between serving the pot roast and the apple pie.

"What does that mean?" I asked.

"I've taken Jesus as my Lord and Savior," she said. "Been saved."

"Saved from what?" I asked.

"Going to hell," she said.

It soon became clear that salvation, by my mother's definition, was unloading one's conscience in front of hundreds of strangers. But mostly it was a concrete set of negative commands: no alcohol should pass our lips; no dancing because hormones might take over; no watching television because of all those bad influences.

Every Sunday, Reverend Chamberlain glared around the sanctuary and accused us in the pews: "Sinners. You are all sinners. You have sinned because you lust." I knew he was looking at me. I had not yet experienced lust, but the way the preacher said it, I knew it had to be bad. Evangelical doctrine taught that, since Eve brought on the wrath of God by being sexual (read: female), the word of God had branded women who desire what feels good and natural as "bad girls." However, it was the Word of God as interpreted by society's rule makers (read: men) with vested interests in constraining women to remain "good girls."

"*Control your urgin', be a virgin. Pet your dog, not your date. Don't be dips, stop at the lips.*"

Mother could not rest until all of the heathens in her family were saved, too, and she was especially determined to convert her husband to her beliefs. My stepfather thought he already was a good Christian. Hadn't he been sprinkled with water? Didn't he attend church regularly and save lives as part of his everyday work? There was no question that he would make it into heaven. He believed more in the miracle of Easter morning than the horrors of Sodom and Gomorrah.

"Methodists are Christian and Missionary Alliances who are allowed to read and think," Dad Browne said one night over dinner. That was the closest my stepfather ever came to denouncing Mother's new church. Before my eyes my mother turned into a dark-tunnel Christian who believed that mankind was inherently corrupt and evil. Sin was absolute. Once Mother "found religion," movies and dancing and sex became taboo subjects. All of a sudden, she was a crusader against young lust. "Look what happened to Emma Bovary," she said. She denied that her physical appetites had ever been satisfied outside of marriage. It was as if all those dates Pat and I went on with Mother had never happened—all those movies where Esther Williams swam and Debbie Reynolds danced. Religion caused a schism in my family that never healed.

It was at a Youth For Christ meeting that I "saw the light." My high school sweetheart, Ken, often studied the Bible with Mother, and then she invited him to go with her to the Billy Graham Crusade in Indianapolis. Was I invited to go along or did I refuse to go? I don't remember. All of a sudden, my boyfriend and my mother were saved, and I was on the outside of the circle. There was a rally held in an old movie theater in Toledo every Saturday evening. An organ played "Old Rugged Cross" and "Just As I Am" and "Amazing Grace" as boys and girls flocked forward and fell on their knees at the altar. Some of them cried, others laughed, as they accepted the promise of entrance into heaven. I wanted that, too, so when Ken gently took my arm and helped me down the aisle, I was ready to be accepted into the enchanted circle.

Chapter Five

⌐ I Solemnly Pledge ⌐

The first time I saw a caduceus it was hanging on the wall of my stepfather's office. In the late 1950s, he was the only general practitioner in Whitehouse, Ohio, a small farming community. The caduceus, that ancient holy symbol of two intertwined serpents, is the emblem of life associated with physical and spiritual health. Because my room was at the top of the stairs, I often heard bits of conversation floating from Dad Browne's office.

"Need to cut out this mole."

"Is it cancer?"

"Won't know until I do the biopsy. Must wait and see."

Perhaps I became a nurse because of seeing Dad Browne's daily devotion to relieving the pain of his patients, observing how his mere presence at her bedside eased an old woman's transition into the next world. Or maybe subconsciously I thought that, by becoming a nurse, I could cure my father, help him return home after his prefrontal lobotomy, something that my mother and the psychiatrists had not been able to achieve.

Barely eighteen, I stood with my classmates, candles lit, proud in our starched caps, dazzling white aprons over blue-checked dresses. We were doing something strangely anachronistic, yet meaningful, as we recited the Nightingale Pledge, an adaptation of the Hippocratic Oath, written in 1893 by Lystra Gretter.

Each night, Florence Nightingale carried a lamp through the hospital she established during the Crimean War. "In that hour of misery, a Lady with a lamp I see," William Wordsworth wrote in his poem "Santa Filomena." Florence ruled her nurses with iron discipline, even locking them up at night to keep them safe from wandering soldiers—or was it to make sure that they showed up in the ward the next morning?

The lobby of Toledo Hospital had the quiet air of a museum with its varnished furniture, waxed floors, and small amplified sounds. However, the medical-surgical floors above conveyed the ambiance of a bus terminal, wheelchairs coming and going on an erratic schedule, people milling about in front of traffic central, the nurses' station. In each room there was a person whose life had been interrupted because an intestine had perforated or a ureter had become blocked by stones. Each wing of the hospital contained a specialty: medical, surgical, gynecology, and obstetrics.

Nursing was many things, but "fun" was not the adjective that sprang to mind. Toledo Hospital School of Nursing was more like entering a religious order than attending an institution of higher learning. Like nuns, my classmates and I wore uniforms that set us apart from the rest of the women our age: blue-and-white-checked dresses with white collars and cuffs on the short sleeves, white shoes, white pantyhose, hemline discreetly below the knee, and white starched caps. We had to be in the dorm by ten thirty every night. Like nuns, we swore to a life of "purity," which translated into no men or alcohol in our rooms, no nail polish, and no heavy makeup. Women who married were forced to leave nurse's training. Like nuns, we were told to follow the orders of a "higher authority," which I quickly learned meant following the orders of doctors. Like nuns, we worked long hours with an occasional "thank you" or "well done" as rewards.

We studied the origin and insertion points of deltoids, pectorals, and trapezius muscles, counted vertebrae and ball-and-socket joints. All of a sudden the heart was the myocardium, the high cheek bone the zygoma. The brain was less prone to daydream when called a cerebellum. There were lists of words with long Latin names to be memorized, the eleven muscles of the thumb, chambers of the heart, classification of diseases of the colon. We learned how lungs exchanged gases, how the heart spun blood around, how kidneys filtered waste. Over and over we were tested on the vocabulary of medicine, words that would forever isolate us from the rest of society. As a true believer in medical progress, I had faith that medical science could erase any mistake.

Along with juggling classes in anatomy, physiology, microbiology, and psychology at Toledo University, we first-year student nurses spent time on the wards. I was assigned to a medical floor for afternoon rounds of medical treatments known as "PM care." This training was designed to help neophyte nurses get used to talking to strangers and touching their skin while taking vital signs and giving backrubs—boot camp for nurses.

"Good evening," I said as I set a fresh decanter of water on the bedside table. Mattie Smith was the name I had written down on the slip of paper. She was eighty and looked small in the oxygen tent enveloping her bed that had kept her alive through many months of advanced emphysema. She looked gray as I peeled back the plastic cocoon to get a better look. The charge nurse was right behind me making rounds. Leaning forward, the charge nurse took the woman's wrist. "This is the way she wanted to go," she said as we removed the oxygen tent and tubes and gave her a new gown. Mattie's limbs were difficult to move, but her lips were curved into a smile.

Becoming a nurse was paying attention to details, knowing which vein to try, knowing that Mr. Lane preferred to lie on his left side with a pillow behind his back and a second one between his legs because that eased the pain in his spine. In our hospital, with its masks of fear and laughter and polished floors and papered feet and gleaming machinery, scalpels parted skin and egos dissolved when confronted by illness or injury. Shock trailed in behind accident victims. Loved ones lay still and breathless behind drawn curtains.

Nursing was an art that took as much skill as a crocheter of lace, each stitch crucial, or the fabric would unravel. A nurse had to be able to read the expression on a patient's face the same way a musician could look at a sheet of music and hear the melody in his or her head, paying attention to heartbeat and oxygen flow day to day, minute to minute. The shadow of death became as real as the radiance of life. Entering the nursing profession meant becoming a minister in the truest sense of the word: the laying on of hands, the wafer under the tongue, the benediction. *"Here is your pain medicine. Now you can rest."*

Rotation meant coming full circle, and my last rotation as a student nurse was the psychiatric affiliation, the same institution where my father had been confined since his lobotomy in 1947. Toledo State Hospital, with its beautiful El Greco faces and gaunt bodies, was a flat, bleak vista, a world hunkered down for a long freeze. Within those walls, human beings were like bumblebees in January, forever stunning themselves against the walls, forever trapped inside their own heads.

Psychiatric nursing was trying to teach people how to take care of themselves—sad, despondent, out-of-touch human beings or people filled with such dizzying energy that they couldn't sit in a chair long enough to eat a meal. Wards were filled with both ends of the spectrum and every personality in between. Keys were the badge of authority, walking through an open door, the most coveted privilege. Dark halls and locked wards. Smoke-filled dayrooms. One-size-fits-all shirts and pants. High-pitched voices. Emotional outbursts. Swaying, staring people who talked to air and then laughed or swore as if they had received answers.

⌒ ⌒

As usual, it was Dad Browne who was there in the parking lot to drive me home after my week of working as a student nurse.

"Let me help you," he said as he lifted my overnight bag and satchel of books into the car. I fell into the front seat beside him. I had homework to do and a case study to write. We drove toward Whitehouse in silence. Always a man of few words, my stepfather taught by example rather than sermons.

"Rough week?" he asked. Smoke swirled up from his pipe.

"Yeah," I replied

"Which ward you working on?" he asked.

"W-2. Chronic schizophrenics," I said. "A room filled with women who don't talk, and so no one talks to them. The nurse in charge told us not to waste too much time feeding each person because we had a whole row of people to feed." The road leading out of the hospital was lined with weeping willows and hardy elms, their leaves lighting up the landscape. "It's hard seeing all those people."

"Sometimes we can't help," Dad Browne said.

"I read my father's chart," I replied.

"Good. I'm glad that you want to know. Things were very different back then. There were no medications for depression. The hospitals were full, and more people were coming back from the war. No one knew what to do with them. Articles appeared in medical journals and in magazines about how lobotomy was going to empty out state hospitals, but of course it didn't work out that way," he said as we pulled into the driveway.

"I'm going to try to see him," I said. From inside, I heard my brother, Charlie, and sister, Barbara, yelling at each other.

"Good," he said as he switched off the ignition. A baby cried, and I wasn't certain which of my two youngest sisters it was—Kathy, who was a toddler the year I had left home, or Jeanne, who was still an infant. Through the office window, I saw an old woman slumped in her chair, patiently waiting the gentle ministrations of my stepfather—just an ordinary evening in the Browne household.

"Good luck on getting some rest," Dad Browne laughed.

Father was on M-8. "I'm here to see Lucien Adams," I said. "I called yesterday."

The nurse consulted her logbook. "Have a seat. I'll fetch him." She came back a few minutes later. "He's in there. Don't sit too close."

She unlocked a door, and I entered the room. There was a wooden table and two chairs and bars on the window. My father sat on the far side of the room. He was tall and his hair was white, his features sallow, his mouth sunken where teeth were missing, his fingers stained by nicotine. He was so thin that a strong wind might have blown him away. The fierce light of intelligence had gone out of his eyes.

"Daddy, it's good to see you." I was four again and waiting for his eyes to light up with recognition. His eyes darted in my direction, then to a spot far to my right. "I'm your daughter." I rose and walked toward him, but stopped. He held his hands up in front of his face, terror in his eyes. "I won't hurt you," I said. He rushed toward me screaming, his hands doubled into fists. A noise erupted, a yowling of pain, the kind a caged animal makes. That was the moment that I understood why the furniture was bolted to the floor and why there were iron bars on the windows. All the teaching of my nursing instructors—no abrupt movements, talk in a calm voice—flew out of my head. I was afraid of this stranger. The father I knew and loved had died long ago but still breathed. I turned and ran out of the building.

Life on a back ward, where the most seriously ill patients were warehoused, was home to my father. Card tables were scattered around the room. A voice ranted from a radio in the corner, but, because of all the noise, it was impossible to hear. Two men jousted in order to root themselves squarely in front of the radio anyway, trying to establish the pecking order—who had the most muscle, the most cunning. Men flitted about, paced, gestured nervously, as if their hands knew a secret sign language. Someone shouted from the corner of the room. There was a fetid odor, like a barnyard full of flies and heat.

"Fuck you," a small, grizzled patient shouted at another man as he walked in front of him. The first man swatted the second, but he was too far away to make contact. A scream erupted. A tall man clutched a younger man's shoulders and shook him, all the while beaming a toothless grin.

The aide took two steps in the direction of the fight, and the instigator slowly released his grip on his prey. Lucien walked to the wall, trying to hide from all the eyes.

"Who wants to play checkers with Lorenzo?" the aide asked. "Anybody? What about you, Lucien?" The aide set out the black and red checkers on a board. Lorenzo was having a deaf day. His hands fluttered in a frenzy of wanting to be understood.

"Don't remember how," Lucien mumbled, but Lorenzo gestured frantically at Lucien to please come and relieve his boredom. Lucien walked slowly to the table and sat down on the edge of the chair.

"Red or black?" the aide asked, as he set up the game. There was the clatter of checker pieces moving on the board. Lorenzo picked at air. "Pay attention. Are you red or black?" Lorenzo pointed at snow falling by the window. "Talk to Lucien, or he won't play."

"Black," Lorenzo whispered as he sat down opposite Lucien.

But Lucien couldn't remember what he was supposed to do with the small, round, red pieces of wood. What was this game they wanted him to play? The aide had placed the red and black pieces on the board, but it made no sense. Colors merged into purple in his brain, too confusing, so he looked at the snow as it piled up on the window sill, simple and pure. Lucien walked to the window and opened it an inch. He stuck a finger through the broken screen.

It was snowing hard, and he breathed in its soft secrets and white lies. Breath was the only private function he had left, the only gentle thing in this asylum with its snow drifts of strait jackets and bandages white as bone. He tapped the window with his icicle finger. Which angel, Michael or Gabriel, would fly through the iron grid and spring him free? When would Christ become a dove swift enough to slip through the vanishing point of the horizon?

Snow collected on the gargoyles and urns. Snow on the iron bars of the windows. Snow on the benches in the courtyard. Snow on the hell of the isolation room and leather straps and electroshock paddles. Snow on the mountain where Abraham raised his icicle-knife against Isaac, under the thumb of the patriarch. Snow on Ruth searching for home and the Virgin Mary looking everywhere for her son. When had faith become this room of ice? Lucien, caught in his scarred body and stammering brain, asked the enigmatic snow for deliverance. No one can touch a man's soul with a knife.

Chapter Six

⌒ LEARNING THE LANGUAGE ⌒

The mossy world of love is as shadowy as a person's deepest self, that soft green bed where fantasy and hope lie down together. Moss has no need to fall, is born fallen, knows how to live in its own light. In my twenties, I didn't know how to say "I need" or "I want;" I didn't believe that I had the right to insist on being heard. A week after I graduated from nurse's training in 1963, I married my high school sweetheart, the president of the local Future Farmers of America, an award-winning drummer, and the son of a farmer-turned-gas-station owner. He was a muscular man with a soft voice and an aquiline nose, and I loved the way his body looked in sunlight.

We met in the Anthony Wayne High School marching band. Ken was a junior and I was a sophomore, a third-chair cornet player. "I saw you, blowing your heart out as you walked toward me, knock knees, pigeon toes and all, and that was it," Ken later said. He asked me out for a date, and I went. I brought him home for dinner to meet my mother and stepfather.

"What are your plans after you finish high school?" my mother asked, flashing a smile as she passed the pot roast and mashed potatoes.

"I want to be a minister," Ken said as he ladled more potatoes onto his already brimming plate. "Marry a minister" was the lesson Pat and I had digested along with our mother's chicken and dumplings.

"How wonderful," Mother said, beaming. "I'd be happy to study the Bible with you, Ken. It would be nice to have someone to discuss the more difficult passages with."

Dad Browne and I exchanged a look. "*What is happening?*" my look asked. "*Don't cause a fuss,*" my stepfather's look said. A couple of weeks later I came home to find Ken and my mother at the dining room table, taking turns reading passages from the Bible: "But as for me, my prayer is unto thee, O Lord, in an acceptable time: O God, in the multitude of thy mercy hear me, in the truth of thy salvation. Deliver me out of the mire…" (Psalms 69, verse 14).

Some of our dates were dipping sheep or raking leaves on the Studer farm ten miles outside of Whitehouse. The farm belonged to Ken's grandparents, with whom Ken and his siblings had lived all their lives. In the Studer household, there were always two sets of parents telling the children what to do. Ken was active in Youth For Christ and preached sermons in many churches. Sometimes Ken and I sang a duet, "How great thou art," he with his strong tenor voice, I with my alto—a proper grooming for a future minister's wife.

Two years later we were sitting in Ken's blue and white Chevrolet eating hamburgers at Burger King. "Will you marry me, Connie?" he asked as he pulled a diamond out of his pocket.

Ken had graduated from Bowling Green State University with a bachelor's degree in sociology and was in his first year at Westminister Theological Seminary in Chestnut Hill, Pennsylvania. We had kissed and petted but had not yet made love. A couple of days after Ken gave me the ring, he left again for school while I was in my third year of nurse's training.

Ken, home for a spring break, stormed into Croxton Hall, the nurses' dormitory, where I was waiting to go out to dinner.

"What's wrong?"

"I just got my grades for last semester. I got a low grade on one of my sermons." His fists were clenched. He went through the front door of the nurses' dorm out to the car. I followed behind. "Where do you want to eat?"

"I've been hungry for a steak all week."

"I can't afford a steak dinner," Ken said as he turned the car onto the highway.

"My treat," I said. "I've earned money picking up extra shifts."

"I don't want steak!" Ken yelled.

"Turn the car around," I said. "I don't need this. I've had a hard week too, as if you cared. I went to see my father on the back ward. He acted like he wanted to hurt me. It was awful. Take me back to Croxton Hall." The rest of the trip was in silence except for my tears. He drove back to the dormitory and stopped at the curb.

"I'm giving this back to you, Ken. I don't think we're ready to get married," I said as I placed the diamond engagement ring on the dashboard.

"What will your mother say?" Ken asked.

"Why are you bringing my mother into this?" I replied. "I still don't know why you and Mother and Charlie went to the Billy Graham Crusade in Chicago six months ago. How did that happen anyway?"

"She asked me if I wanted to go and I did," he said. "She went with Charlie and me to the front when we were saved. Are you jealous of your mother?"

"Get over yourself," I replied. "I need a break from you and all your dramas."

"Fine. Have it your way," he said as he roared away.

As children, Pat and I had accompanied our mother on her dates after she divorced my father. There was the man whom she had met at a local Friday night dance. There was the married man where she worked. Mother had amber hair and charm and knew how to show off her assets to their best advantage. She missed the adrenaline rush of desire, saw her daughters growing up and entering new lives of sex, entering professions, and having money of their own. All those endless possibilities while she was stuck in a marriage that was coming apart at the seams.

There were many phone calls and letters of apology from Ken in the next months. When he came home for Christmas vacation, he asked me to marry him again, and I accepted a second time. We were married in the Whitehouse Methodist Church, the same church where my father had been a pastor so many years before. By that time he had been confined in Toledo State Hospital for sixteen years. Candlelight shone in the chapel's bejeweled windows as we walked down the aisle. Watching from the pews were aunts, uncles, the cynical, the twice-divorced, and the silver-anniversary celebrants. I repeated the words after the minister, about loving and obeying, believing that love was like clouds moving across the skin, allowing sun warmth to penetrate. I didn't know that just as suddenly the warmth could slip away.

Married less than a month, my husband and I settled into our apartment in Chestnut Hill, Pennsylvania. I was twenty, a newly minted registered nurse, and employed full-time on the evening shift at a local hospital. I worked on an Isolation Ward, where patients with staphylococcal infections and tuberculosis knew the loneliness of being set apart as entities to be feared. After six months, I transferred to a brand new Intensive Care Unit. For me, ICU always meant "I See You; I am paying attention; I will watch over you to make sure you are safe."

I still had not learned the language of grief the night our phone rang. Ken was studying for an Old Testament exam, and on one of my nights off from work, I sat reading *War and Peace.*

"Daddy's died," Pat said.

"How?"

"They said a heart attack," she replied. "Found him in a chair on the ward at Toledo State Hospital. Would you go with me to the funeral?"

The silence became uncomfortable. All I could think of was the last time I saw my father, when he had yelled and lunged at me. There was also the nursing job that I had just started, leaving my husband of four months, and not enough money in our savings account for even a warm winter coat, let alone money for a trip half way across the country. All valid excuses, but not the real reason I didn't attend my father's funeral. I had no words to say what was in my heart.

"I can't leave," I said. "Won't Mama go with you?"

"She says it wouldn't be proper for her to go," Pat replied.

"Why?" I asked.

"I'm not sure, but I think it's because she divorced Daddy. Or maybe it's because she never took us to see our father's relatives. They're strangers," Pat said, her voice breaking.

"Can't Dave go with you?" I asked.

"He's got a wedding to do that day. It's okay. I'll go alone."

"What is it?" Ken asked after I got off the phone.

"That was Pat," I said. "Our father died. Pat wanted me to go to the funeral with her, but I can't. I just started my job, and they won't understand if I leave now."

"And there's no money," Ken said.

"That, too," I said.

After the funeral, Pat sent me a long letter. "Daddy looked nice but much older than his fifty-four years. Delnoe, Daddy's brother, has a good sense of humor and is tall and gangly and reminded me of our father. His wife Muriel told me that a long time ago Delnoe and Daddy were discussing how they thought children should be raised. Delnoe said he was going to tell his children the truth. Daddy said he wasn't. He was going to tell his children a lot of lovely lies.

"Daddy's sister, Mildred, said that none of the family ever held it against Mama for divorcing Daddy. They all knew that she worked hard, right alongside Daddy in the church work. They all agreed that Mama did the right thing in building a new life for herself and us after the doctors gave up hope of Daddy's ever recovering after the lobotomy. They told me that Daddy almost died of rheumatic fever when he was seventeen. There were about forty people at the funeral. Here is part of the obituary: 'Lucien Kellog Adams, fifth child of Kellog P. and Bessie E. Adams, was born near Harlem, Ohio on January 25, 1910 and died at Toledo, Ohio on July 16, 1964. It is his spirit which remains in the memory of his family and friends. A joyous, optimistic, driving spirit which found an outlet in church activities, in poetry and the dramatic arts. It was a noble spirit. May it rest in peace.' Some funerals are graduation ceremonies. All my love, Your sister, Pat."

Many more years would pass before I was able to admit that my father had died in a mental institution. In spite of my nursing education, the social stigma of mental illness was stronger than the love I felt for my father. How brave my sister was to attend our father's funeral alone, to meet our Adams relatives for the first time.

⌒ ⌒

Learning the language of love was hard work, requiring concentration and discipline and commitment. How a glance, a turn of the head, or a touch could say more than words. I believed that once my husband achieved his education, we would light in one place and build a home like everyone else.

"My professor wants me to apply for a scholarship that the Dutch government gives to foreign students," Ken said one Sunday morning as he sipped his coffee. In order to save money, we had moved out of our two-room apartment into student housing that the seminary provided. We now lived in one large room, with a curtain dividing the sleeping area from the sitting/eating area. We shared a kitchen and bath with four other student families. Children ran up and down the hall outside our room, their laughter filtering through the walls.

"Holland?" I asked. "How will going to Holland help you become a minister?"

"I want to get my doctorate," he said. "Maybe teach in an university."

"That's the first I've heard about this," I replied. "You always said you were going to be a minister."

"My professors don't think I'm cut out for it," he said. "I don't think so either."

"Why?" I asked.

"People get on my nerves," he replied.

Six months later we arrived in Amsterdam, a long way from rural Ohio where we grew up, and even farther in spirit from anywhere we had ever been. Amsterdam, the city of

Rembrandt and Spinoza, the philosopher who was branded a heretic because he said God and nature were synonymous. The city where Anne Frank, hidden away in an attic, wrote, "In spite of everything, I know men are good." Even though the small country had been overridden by Hitler and had been drowned more than once by sea water, the Netherlands always managed to remain a land of fertile soil and fair cities, a peaceful and tolerant nation, where faiths could mingle, Mennonite and Catholic, Protestant and Jew, the lion lying down with the lamb.

Amsterdam looked like a pop-up city of narrow houses plunked down on skinny streets of dreams. Rows of cafes and bicycles choked toy streets. Bells rang from handlebars and church towers. Houseboats bobbed on their anchors as they lined the canals. It was 1965 when Ken and I lugged our steamer trunk up a narrow, spiraling staircase, past the portraits of our landlord's ancestors, up to our two rooms on the third floor. Our living space was a room with sunflower wallpaper, two rattan chairs, a table, and a window that opened out to a small balcony. Between smokestacks, I caught a glimpse of sunlight dancing off the *Ijselmeer*. The bedroom was large enough for only a bed and a slanted ceiling with a skylight that opened to the stars. With another tenant, we shared a bathroom and an alcove with a hotplate that served as a kitchen.

While still in the United States, we had purchased a Dutch grammar book and quizzed each other on vocabulary words and laughed at each other's wild pronunciations. Walking down *Vrijheidslaan*, we took in the barrage of Dutch consonants. Amsterdam was a United Nations of accents. Walking in any direction, it was possible to hear German, Dutch, Italian, and Scandinavian. Music was in the bicycle bells, the toot of the tram horn, and the organ grinder's repetitious ditties—"*lang zal ze leven, lang zal se leven…*" The air smelled of *nasi goreng*, poached salmon, and coffee thick with cream. Hucksters in open-air stalls begged us to buy their apples and pears. We walked past hippies throwing Frisbees to their dogs, past the *Rosseburt* where women, wearing only bras and panties, sat on display in large windows, waiting for patrons. The odor of marijuana wafted out of cafes. Government-issued porta-potties dotted city parks to accommodate street people. The Dutch, true to their core belief in pragmatism and tolerance, embraced the rule of "the sovereignty of one's own domain." "Live and let live" was their creed.

Twice a week we bicycled to a small room in the basement of the university library and studied the Dutch language. Unlike American universities, *Vrije Universiteit* had no central campus but consisted of buildings scattered all over Amsterdam. In *Taal Practicum*, our long-suffering instructor laid out the rules of the Dutch language: "There are two forms for 'the,' *de* and *het*, depending upon whether the following noun is masculine or feminine. Adjectives take the ending 'e' before singular and plural nouns of both genders."

"Say 'it's going to rain' in Dutch," Jan said.

My tongue stuck to the top of my palate as I stumbled over the words. "*Het gaat regenen.*" Jan corrected my pronunciation, the smoothness of his language running over mine.

My brain was tired from all the new nouns and verbs and rules and long words ending with "g's" and "sch's" that were supposed to explode from the back of the throat, as if you were spitting out phlegm. However, Ken and I gradually understood the clerk in the bakery, and he understood us when we asked for a half loaf of wheat bread. The street where we lived, *Ooievaarsweg,* meant Stork Street. Finally, we could carry on a conversation with our landlord, Meneer DeZwaart, a diminutive Buddha, bald and pink and portly, and his apple-cheeked, energetic wife. It was Mevrouw who explained the custom of buying fresh meat and milk daily. *"Het is gezellig,"* Mevrouw said. And the day arrived when Dutch sentences tripped off our tongues: *"Waar is je fiets?"* (Where is your bicycle?) *"Wat idioot!"* (How ridiculous!) *"Waar dank je aan?"* (What are you thinking of?) And I finally learned that *gezellig* meant to be sociable, cozy, at home.

In my twenties, I thought love was following my husband wherever his academic ambitions took him and working double shifts at the hospital in order to keep food in the cupboard and coal in the furnace. Love was learning Dutch and pedaling twenty minutes in the rain to work at the *Luthersche Deakonessen Inrichting* in a blue dress and white apron and stiff white cap, a uniform that looked very much like what I had worn as a student nurse. I helped get patients ready for *ontbijt,* a simple breakfast of bread with cheese or strawberries on top, with tea or coffee. All the nurses trooped downstairs for breakfast, recited a prayer over the loudspeaker, then trooped back upstairs for the usual routine of preparing patients for surgery, passing medications, and changing dressings. With the Netherlands' humane approach to health care, no one, not even foreign students like my husband and me, were turned away. Universal health care was seen as a right instead of a privilege bestowed only on those blessed with money.

Love was entering a hospital ward full of men and answering their questions about why the United States was in Vietnam, while giving them baths and medications. "What right does America have to impose its form of government on them?" a man asked.

"There was a race riot in Selma," the man in the next bed said. "Why do you Americans insist on killing each other?" And I felt bereft, as if I would never be able to return home again. I was forced to look at my country of origin through the eyes of my Dutch patients and to question what I saw reflected there. That was what opened my mind to questioning all of my previous beliefs as well, about my mother's increasingly controlling personality, about what ambitions I had for my own life, and about how I deserved respect from my husband.

⮑ ⮐

I had grown up hearing the story in Genesis about how God created Eve out of Adam's rib: "And they were both naked and they were not ashamed." Since she was an intelligent woman, Eve wanted knowledge and wanted her share of the apple, but God said, "Eat of it and you shall surely die." Eve had a mind of her own; Eve saw that the tree was good for food and that it was pleasant to the eyes. I was raised to believe that if a wife supported her husband in his educational and professional ambitions, all would be well. It only dawned on me several years into our marriage that I had a right to similar ambitions.

"I want to take classes," I told my husband as we began our second year in Amsterdam. We had saved enough money for me to quit my nursing position at the *Luthersche Deakonessen Inrichting.* The scholarship from the Dutch government had come through for our second year. Ken was well on his way to earning his *doctorandus,* the residence work towards a doctorate. We had visited the *Rijksmuseeum,* the art museum displaying Dutch masterpieces by Rembrandt and Vermeer. We had wandered for hours through the *Stedelijkjmuseeum,* past paintings of Rauschenberg and Matisse and Van Gogh. Two rooms were not difficult to keep clean.

"What classes to do you want to take?" he asked.

"English literature," I said.

"You came to Holland to study English literature?"

"I came to Holland so that you could work on your doctorate. I have always wanted to study English literature."

Because the first-year Dutch students believed in starting at the root of their field of study and working forward, I found myself studying Anglo-Saxon and Old English. I attended the lectures in Dutch, translated them into English to make sure I understood the meaning, and then translated it back into Dutch in order to participate in class. The Dutch students didn't know what to make of me, a quiet, skinny woman who only knew what she was going to say long after the banter was over. The stranger with the long brown hair always hovering on the fringe. A woman in a foreign land, studying a foreign language, that was the ancestor of her native tongue.

At night the balcony was where I escaped to be alone, to watch how the *Ijselmeer* exhaled its chill breath into the air. As fog cleared, the moon slid out from behind a cloud and shone on the rows of gabled houses lining *Ooievaarsweg.* Their windows glowed sightlessly in the moonlight. A breeze rustled and creased the water like satin. Amsterdam was a grand dowager gazing into her looking glass. One could forgive vanity in a lady so regal.

"Connie, what are these?" Ken yelled as he stuck his face out of the window. He held out the cloth bag that Dutch women used to carry home their purchases. When he turned it upside down, four coffee spoons fell out.

"Little coffee spoons, *lepeltjes,*" I replid. "They're only stainless steel. I thought it would be nice to have them when my mother and sisters come for their visit."

Against my stepfather's wishes, my mother had embarked on two large trips with my little sisters in tow. They had spent ten days in the Far East, and on their next tour, they would be in Amsterdam. They were planning to visit Ken and me in our tiny rooms. I was nervous about how my mother would react to our sparse living conditions.

"We can't afford these," my husband said, as he threw them at my back. I was too stunned to respond. Much later I knew what I should have said: "*It's my working at the* Luthersche Deakonessen Inrichting *that gives me the right to buy four little spoons if I want to. I'm the one that worked in a hospital back in the states so that you could finish seminary.*" I still believed that if I helped my husband achieve his dreams, that someday we would have a home and be able to go out for dinner and a movie like everyone else. My husband could never relax, never believed it was okay to laugh and play once in a while. From that incident on, my marriage became a state of constant vigilance, instead of a soft place to fall.

My mother and little sisters arrived for their four-day visit. Ken and I introduced them to raw herring and to *hagelslag,* chocolate sprinkles that the Dutch put on bread. We took them to the Anne Frank house and to Edam and for a canal ride. While navigating Amsterdam's busy streets, Jeanne ran out in front of a tram. Ken pulled her to safety just in time.

"That was close," Ken said as he held Jeanne in his arms.

"I'd never be able to go home again if anything happened to these girls," Mother said, visibly shaken. "Their father didn't want to let them come on this trip. We had a big fight about it, but I won."

Even though Ken and I had lived far away from my parents' home in Whitehouse, Ohio, ever since we were married, the stories that filtered back to us made it clear that my parents were fighting often over Barbara's dating habits, which ended with her becoming pregnant and marrying right out of high school. Charlie, drunk and speeding, was driving Dad Browne's car when he and a buddy were involved in a terrible accident. Always there was the old fight of Dad Browne's leniency and my mother's firm discipline. Neighbors had walked in and had seen my mother and brother exchanging blows. Pat told me that when she and Dave visited, they heard our mother and Barbara fighting. I was grateful that my husband and I lived far away.

We went back to our tiny rooms. Mother never asked about how Ken and I were doing in this foreign land or about the classes I was taking. The next day my mother and little sisters rejoined their tour as they headed to Italy, then to England.

By the end of our second year in Holland, Ken had completed the residence work toward his doctorate and was awarded a *doctorandus* degree. In a picture commemorating this day, Ken and I stood in a park, along with his three professors. Ken held his diploma while I smiled proudly at him, my long hair swept up into an intricate knot at the back of my head like a proper Dutch matron.

When Ken sent out his resume for teaching positions in the United States, he received an offer from Illinois College, a private liberal arts institution with a reputation for academic excellence. Ken and I pored over the atlas trying to learn more about the city and state that would be our new home. The campus had a rolling green lawn and tall elms and brick buildings that had stood since 1829.

Ken took the position as instructor in sociology. My eyes lit up when he told me that one of his benefits was that family members of faculty could attend college tuition-free. I enrolled for courses and was granted permission to use Dutch as my foreign language. A professor at Calvin College agreed to take me on as his student. I read ten Dutch books, wrote papers on them, and then traveled to Calvin College for an oral exam. Like a circus performer, I juggled roles—faculty wife, full-time student, and college nurse—and often had trouble keeping all three balls in the air.

"My parents called today," Ken said one evening as we both studied. The only heat in the farmhouse we rented came from a space heater in the living room. "They don't know what to do with Kathy. They asked if we'd let her stay with us. She thinks she wants to attend college here." Kathy was Ken's youngest sister, a tiny, quiet girl, whom I barely knew. We both had sisters named Kathy.

"I've got all I can handle, and then some," I said.

"My parents are desperate," he replied. "Kathy has had some serious psychological problems. They're worried about depression. I told them we'd try to help."

"You said that without asking me?"

"I couldn't say 'no' to my parents."

"You're going to have to help me with her," I said. "Promise?"

"I promise."

A few days later we were loading up our car for a trip back to Whitehouse, Ohio, for Thanksgiving with my family when the phone rang.

"He's crazy," Mother yelled into the phone.

"Who's crazy?" I thought we had a bad connection.

"Your stepfather threw me and your little sisters out of the house!" she cried. "All of my clothes were on the lawn!"

"What happened?" I asked.

"We had a terrible fight over him giving Charlie money all the time, and he's still angry that I took Kathy and Jeanne on those long trips."

"Where are you now?"

"In the apartment above the garage. I called the police. He belongs in the State Hospital. He's crazy."

"You can't mean that. Don't do anything until we get there."

"It's already done," Mother said.

"What do you mean?" I yelled, but Mother had already hung up.

Ten hours later Ken and I pulled into the driveway of my parents' home. The house that had remained standing through more than half a century of sub-zero winters and late fall tornadoes was now being tested by my parents' fights. The house was dark when we entered. I found Dad Browne standing in the bathroom, shirtless, removing more than a three-day shadow from his face.

"What in the world happened?"

"I couldn't take it anymore," he said as he spread on more shaving cream and moved the razor over his upper lip, flicking off the excess foam into the sink. "Nothing I do is ever good enough for her. I give up." His face looked gray under the fluorescent light. His hand shook as he wielded the razor. "She called the police on me. Said she'd have me put in Toledo State Hospital, but the police didn't agree. I told them that if they took me, they'd have to take her, too, because she was more violent than I was. I don't know if we can continue like we are."

"What about Kathy and Jeanne?" My little sisters were ten and eleven years old.

His face softened and he slumped forward, a sign of resignation more eloquent than words. For the next few days, Ken and I tried to establish some sort of communication between my parents. Ken went up to talk to my mother in the apartment above the garage while I tried to comfort my stepfather. Then Ken and I huddled to talk about strategy and switched places in an effort to restore some semblance of peace. Thanksgiving found Ken and me in a local diner eating turkey sandwiches.

When Ken had to return to Illinois to teach, I stayed on in the house with my stepfather. Clearly, my mother saw me as choosing my stepfather's side, but I saw myself more as a courier risking life and limb by carrying messages into enemy territory. Mother was a general marshalling her troops. Dad Browne had the look of a just-released prisoner of war, haggard but relieved to find himself wounded but still alive.

"Tell me about your service in World War II. Were you hurt?" I asked. We sat in the living room where my mother had set out her souvenirs from her trips to the Far East and Europe: dolls from India, silver spoons from Belgium, a plastic replica of the Eiffel Tower.

"I got a purple heart, but it had nothing to do with bravery," he said, forever humble. "My roommate was cleaning his gun in the tent. It went off, and I got a bullet in my leg." He told me how sad he was when his first wife died of cancer and how happy they had been when they adopted Barbara and Charlie as babies. "I really do love your mother," he said as tears gathered in his eyes. "She just makes me so angry sometimes."

"I know. Do you want to go to church tomorrow?" My family's crisis had kept all the small town tongues busy. The Methodist Church, of which Dad Browne was a pillar, had become a symbol of everything wrong in his second marriage.

"If you hadn't gone with me to church last Sunday, I'd never have been able to step into that church again," my stepfather told me a week later as he drove me back to my home in Illinois. Mother had rented a house for herself and my little sisters. Dad Browne courted her all over again, and six months later, they again lived under one roof, but only after bitter negotiations that ended in a signed agreement.

When Ken's sister came to live with us, I reluctantly assumed the role of surrogate mother to a very depressed child. I had all the responsibility of feeding her and helping her with her college assignments and listening when her heart was broken by her latest beau, but none of the authority to make parental decisions. When she got failing grades in some of her classes, there was a huge fight between Ken and his sister.

"You are embarrassing me," he told Kathy. "Straighten up or I'll send you back home."

Kathy ran crying outside and ran down the road. Ken ran after her and pulled her physically back in the house. This situation was clearly out of control.

"I'm going to call the school psychologist," I said to Kathy. "The only way I'll let you live with us is if you get some help."

"I'll be glad to go, but Ken needs to go too," Kathy said.

"How would that look? Everybody on campus would know," he said.

Everything came to a crashing conclusion in the spring of 1971. Ken was told that his contract would not be renewed at Illinois College unless he finished his doctorate, sending my husband's stress level through the roof.

"I need to go back to Holland, to be near my professors, in order to write my dissertation," Ken said. The dissertation was the big black gorilla peering into our bedroom window every night. I still fantasized that once Ken had his doctorate, there would be peace in our home and a chance to enjoy life.

"I'm pregnant," I said. Eight years into our marriage, I really thought I couldn't get pregnant, then this miracle. Ken's side of the bed was silent. "Did you hear me?"

"I heard you," he said. "We really do have to go back to Amsterdam. That's the only way for me to get the dissertation done."

"What about money?" I asked. "I won't be able to work, with the baby and all."

"We'll have to use our savings," he replied. "We can sell our furniture."

"What about Kathy?" I asked.

"It'll be a good excuse for her to go back home," Ken said. "I can't tell my parents we don't want her here."

That spring I received my bachelor's degree in English literature from Illinois College. I was able to complete my degree in two years because some credits from nurse's training were applicable. I was given credit for the Anglo-Saxon and Old English classes I had taken at *Vrije Universiteit* in Amsterdam. Kathy went home to the Studer farm. Ken and I sold our table and chairs and sofa and bed and prepared to return to the Netherlands once again.

I wasn't quite ready to admit to myself that married love should not be a sliver under my fingernail that I had to endure no matter how badly my finger bled—that obedience and love were not the same thing. That sex was physiological and biochemical while love should be a two-way commitment, agapé rather than eros, or it wouldn't endure. Words emerge from lips and vocal cords when the brain is ready to form them and the heart is able to hear. I have always been a slow learner, but I do get there in the end.

Chapter Seven

⇐ LILITH'S DAUGHTER COMES HOME ⇒

When does mother-love begin? At conception? At the first sign of movement? Or when the baby finally snuffles for milk at his mother's breast? *Mater.* Mistress of the World. Ruler of the Womb. Mother, the one who carries new life beneath her heart, a heavy burden, new life she'll help through scraped knees and measles and wounds, both real and imaginary.

The second time my husband and I landed in Amsterdam, I was seven months pregnant. The air was fragrant with tulips and sea breeze, just as I had remembered. Holland still struggled to maintain its uneasy truce between land and water. Amsterdam still was a city of narrow houses with gingerbread-and-icing gables. *Spiegelstraat* translated as Street of Mirrors. *Bloemenmarkt,* a flower market, fragrant with tulips and roses, floated on barges along the *Singel. Westerstraat* was lined with cafes decorated in cozy shades of brown. Cafes signified what was best about Dutch culture: allowing people to talk while others listened, to be made welcome, to politely disagree, and to make room for everyone, even foreigners like my husband and me.

"People who close their curtains have something to hide" was the Dutch belief. We lived in a hotel for over a month, and as we walked the streets of Amsterdam looking for lodging, I was jealous of the husband framed in the window ladling out potatoes and the wife cutting up meat for their smiling daughter.

"Illinois College won't renew my contract unless I finish my doctorate," Ken had said one evening at dinner in our Jacksonville home a few weeks after I had told him that we had a baby on the way. It was 1971, and American universities were full of protesters. Four students were about to die at Kent State. The war in Vietnam was at its height. The first Earth Day had just been held. I agreed to return to the Netherlands, because I still believed that, once my husband earned his doctorate, we would have a home like everyone else. Home was always the next place after this one, a tantalizing mirage just out of reach.

Our Amsterdam home was two rooms we rented from an elderly lady who promised she was going south for the winter. She never went, so we shared our kitchen and bathroom with her. Each morning, my husband went to an office at the *Vrije Universiteit* to work on his thesis, while I read and knitted and prepared for the birth of our child. Dutch friends came bearing baby clothes, visibly perplexed why Ken and I had chosen to return to Holland to have our baby.

Pregnancy, that nine-month odyssey through inner space. And I cried. Blame it on hormones or maybe not. I wept for the little girl who wasn't afraid to swing on a rope from one haymow to another. I wept for the safety of my stepfather's brownstone house and for the cherry pie my mother used to bake. I wept because I was lonely for friends and family back home. I wept because of the swelling in my ankles and the heartburn that erupted whenever I lay on my back. I wept because the woman I saw in the mirror in the maternity smock wasn't the woman I thought I had become. One moment I was Earth Mother and the next the Wicked Witch of the West.

"You haven't gained enough weight," the Dutch doctor told me at my eight-month exam. "I want to see you again in a week. If you don't put on more weight, we'll have to hospitalize you."

A few days later, I was awakened by pain. My water broke in the bathroom. "Call the ambulance," I yelled to Ken.

"The baby's too early," he said.

"Don't argue." Within minutes, the ambulance carried me to the *Vrije Universiteit Ziekenhuis.* As a student nurse, I had helped deliver many babies but had no understanding of what "natural childbirth" felt like, how becoming a mother meant the painful reality of tissues expanding, cartilage stretching, cervix dilating.

"Don't scream. You won't have energy to push," a voice in my ear said as my fingernails chewed up Ken's palm. My legs rode high in the stirrups. Green leggings hung down like chaps. "*Push.*" As if I had a choice. Six hours later, our son was laid on my chest, still flecked with the blood of arrival. They cut the umbilical cord. "Well done," my husband said, with a kiss.

Back in my room, I slept, and then they brought my son to me. His spirit gave me hope that any dream was possible. His early arrival meant he was a lightweight, not quite six pounds. I unwrapped him, counted his fingers and toes, studied the face that I would come to know very well. His eyes flashed and squinted. His arms rose and sank in wavelike motions, as if he were conducting some unheard, ancient music. My breasts grew heavy with milk. With each look, each coo, each touch, my son rewired me. Within minutes, motherhood was an immutable fact, as much a part of my DNA as my brown hair and eyes. The woman I was before that day was as insignificant as a dream.

Ken left every morning to work on his thesis, and once a month, Chris and I strolled to the Well Baby Clinic provided by the Dutch government. Chris thrived on breast milk, quickly gaining weight. As he lay on the table, I kissed his neck, feet, ribs, the powdery skin creases while he kicked and waved. His chicken-like cries of hunger diminished to grunting and smacking as he found my breast.

"How is your thesis coming?" I asked Ken.

"Not well," he said, and I knew better than to inquire further. One night, two months after my son's birth, Ken and our landlady were in the kitchen. I heard angry voices and pans hitting the sink. Police appeared at the door. The landlady accused Ken of threatening her. She agreed not to press charges if we moved in the morning. We were on the phone long into the night trying to find shelter. For the first time, I understood how my mother felt when, after my father went into Toledo State Hospital, we were forced to leave the Whitehouse Methodist parsonage. Fear that my baby and I might end up on the street became as real as a looming train wreck.

We moved three times the year my son was born. Like a turtle, I dragged home with me wherever we went. We sublet an apartment from university students who were taking a two-month hiatus from their studies. When they returned, we moved again.

"We need to cash your traveler's checks," Ken said one night at dinner. A shred of lettuce stuck to his lip. I watched, fascinated, how it perched there while he talked.

"No. That's all I have in case Chris and I need to get back to the States," I said, bracing myself against what was coming.

"Don't do this." He reached across the table and grabbed my wrist.

"Those checks are my only security." I froze, not knowing whether I should expect a blow. "Let go of my wrist."

Ken began sending out his resumé for jobs at universities in the United States, without success. He applied for grants. I didn't know where we would land next, but through it all I hung onto my sweet son. It quickly became clear that Chris had a wide emotional repertoire: he sighed with pleasure, ranted with loneliness, laughed when breeze ruffled his blond hair, and cooed over a favorite toy. Then there were those times when we disagreed: I welcomed his nap time, but he didn't. I thought his cereal would hit the spot in his hungry stomach. He preferred it on the floor.

He was eight months old when we came home to America.

I grew up hearing the creation story as it appeared in Genesis, how Eve was the first woman created from Adam's rib, and because she tempted Adam and initiated him into the mysteries of the garden, God cast them from Eden. Much later I learned that the book of Genesis contained two separate and mutually contradictory accounts of the Creation. According to Jewish scholars, Lilith was Adam's first wife, fashioned from the dust of the Earth by the Lord Almighty in the same second that Adam also breathed for the first time. Lilith was a rebellious woman portrayed as part snake and part bird, "the winding serpent who is Lilith." She was a woman who wanted equal billing in the Creation story, and when she didn't get it, she had no recourse but to flee.

Although Lilith was demonized by early Jewish culture as a symbol of promiscuity and disobedience, I prefer to think of Lilith as the first woman who knew she deserved equality with her man. Those who believed that Eve sprang from Adam's rib called God *Yahweh*, "storm god." Those who thought the first woman sprang from clay called God *Elohim*, "mountain god." Perhaps Lilith was the original divinity, female, life-giving, the source of all creation, a lady who lived in the midst of a tree.

"I can't live like this anymore," I told Ken soon after we returned to the United States in the summer of 1972. He had accepted a fellowship that paid three thousand dollars a year at Cornell. My nursing registration was still in Illinois, and the New York nursing accreditation office maintained that, because of a backlog, it might take over a year to obtain a nursing license. There was nothing to be done except get any job I could. I worked full-time typing Thai and Japanese phonetics—languages I didn't read or speak, gibberish. However, the money from the job kept food on the table and paid the rent for the year that we lived in Ithaca, the year after our son was born. I was heartsick.

"I'm going to move to Boulder, Colorado," I told him. "Chris is coming with me."

"Why Boulder?" He paced up and down the living room.

"The summer we were there at the University of Colorado was the best three months of our marriage. You were happy with your anthropology institute, and I was happy taking American literature classes. I fell in love with the mountains."

"How are you going to live?" he asked.

"I've got my nursing registration in Colorado, and I've got an appointment for an interview for a position at Boulder Community Hospital the day after we get in Boulder. I've never had trouble getting a job," I said.

"This is true," he said softly, rocking our son in his arms.

For months, I had been packing up Chris' toys and clothes and dishes and a rocker that my stepfather had given me. Even though boxes accumulating in the corner of the living room were a constant reminder that I was planning to leave, Ken did not believe I would really do it until the final month.

"Come talk to her, Dave," I heard him say into the phone. "She's going to take Chris and move to Colorado. Thanks," he said and hung up.

"Why'd you call Dave?" I asked.

"I thought, since he was a minister, he could talk some sense into you," Ken said.

"It's too late for counseling, especially from my brother-in-law," I replied. "If you'd have gone with me to a therapist when we first got back to the States, maybe it would've helped. I'm ashamed how we're living. That I had to wean Chris from breast milk when he was only eight months old so that he could go to a babysitter because I had to work. That I'm typing and typing every day in order to keep food on our table. That we haven't lived long enough in one place for me to have a stable nursing position. I'm tired of worrying that any way the wind blows we're going to be pulled somewhere else."

My sister and brother-in-law arrived ten hours later and a marathon, last-ditch counseling session began. Dave talked to me, then to Ken, and then I sat in the car with Pat while Dave told Ken that I was serious about leaving. It was as if it were all new information that Ken was hearing. For three years I had tried to tell him that we needed to have a home and a support system of friends and a home church, but my words had not made an impression. When Pat and Dave left a few hours later, my husband finally realized that our marriage was over.

It was raining the day in July, 1973, when I left my husband. Chris was eighteen months old. At the last moment, I had called my sister, Pat, and asked her if she would like to go on a trip.

"Where are you going?" she asked.

"Boulder, Colorado," I whispered, as if saying the words would make a new home real. Rocky Mountains would appear outside my window instead of the concrete buildings of

Cornell. The last day Ken and I were together was peaceful, like the stillness of a hospital room after the resuscitation team has done its best and loved ones come to kiss the dearly departed good-bye. Ken helped me load the U-Haul that was attached to the car. We kissed without saying a word. Ken placed Chris in his car seat. As I pulled out of the driveway, I looked back. Ken stood in the driveway staring, then turned on his heels and walked back to the apartment.

Once on the highway headed west from Ithaca, it began to rain. The windshield wipers whispered: *heartsick"* and *"wanderlust,"* as they went back and forth. Rain fell on cars as they moved slowly ahead, behind, alongside. Chris slept in his car seat, his left cheek resting on the padded bar. I drove past houses with boarded-up windows, caved-in porch steps, yards overgrown with thistles and dandelions and tumbleweed. Hundreds of miles passed without a sign of a gas station or even a horse grazing. When I opened the glove compartment, there was a note, "I love you. Ken." There were notes in the picnic basket of sandwiches, notes in Chris' diaper bag, notes in the trunk of the car. The road west passed yellow houses with wide porches, hay fields where bales were stacked like giant pillows, small towns the size of Whitehouse, and university towns the size of Ithaca. At a filling station, I threw away Ken's notes and felt sorry for him, because he still didn't know that love meant having a peaceful, warm home with enough nourishment to sustain everyone under its roof. Love was thinking more about the other person than yourself. I was a slow learner when it came to speaking up for myself; it took a long time for my heart and vocal cords to learn the words I needed to say.

We arrived at my sister and brother-in-law's Ohio home late in the afternoon. Call it synchronicity or serendipity, but my mother, stepfather, and two youngest sisters were visiting Pat and Dave. They were in the backyard having a picnic.

"You're on your way to Colorado?" Dad Browne asked.

"Yes. That's where Chris and I need to be," I replied.

"I understand." With those two words, I knew that I had his blessing. A picture from that day showed my stepfather holding my baby son on his lap. Then Chris put out his hand to pet a puppy, a look of rapture lighting his face.

"But Ken is such a good Christian," was all my mother said. In her mind, going forward and accepting salvation so many years before at the Billy Graham Crusade exempted my husband from any other transgressions during the intervening years.

How could I explain to my family how the air in the three rooms I had shared with my husband had gotten wet and gray and heavy as fog? How I had beaten eggs in a bowl and watched myself beating eggs but couldn't remember what I was planning to do with them. I had combed my hair and never felt the plastic teeth touch my scalp. Making the bed, I had leaned over to tuck in the sheets and had collapsed in slow motion on the half-made bed and then jumped up, afraid that I would never be able to rise again. I couldn't explain how air in the house had turned into water and I had been in danger of drowning. The last week in Ithaca, I had smelled change coming with the lilac buds and maple leaves and freshly mowed grass.

The atlas was spread out on the front seat of the car between Pat and me. "Start out from where you are this moment, and then let the map lead you somewhere you've never been," my stepfather had instructed during one of our driving lessons. This moment my sister was reading *Five Smooth Stones* out loud to me, and my son was sleeping peacefully in his seat behind me. The rain had stopped. A river glittered between the trees. The car ahead of us bore the bumper sticker: "Never drive faster than your angels can fly."

Like Lilith, I had fled my marriage, and at the end of my journey lay so many unknowns. Would I find a nursing position? Would I be able to find a competent babysitter for my son? I had made an intuitive leap, and the logic came later. I had tapped into a whole other reality that couldn't be reached by intellect or by following a road map or by linear thinking. That night when we slept in a motel, I dreamt of a house with a yard where my son and I would plant lilacs and petunias. Sunlight would illuminate cottonwoods and reflect gently off aspen trees. Our home would provide cool water from the tap, warmth from the fireplace, and cupboards full of nourishment. Love would no longer make me cry. Like Lilith, my soul knew what it needed just as thirst knew water and hunger knew bread.

Chapter Eight

⌖ INSCAPE ⌖

The last night my husband and I slept under the same roof, I cooked orange roughy and baked potatoes, and afterwards, I stood at the sink washing dishes, muttering "This is the last time I'll wash his dishes" under my breath. As I slept on the couch, the room grew huge, as if I were looking through the wrong end of a telescope at my life. Here I was at the end of my marriage with the map I had always used in my hand, but nothing was recognizable. I could no longer put a dot on the map and say, "This is where I am, this is where I'm going." Fear mingled with grief that our marriage was over. No trust, no love, that simple. However, leaving a marriage is never simple, because it is the death of a dream.

When my son and I arrived in Colorado in the summer of 1973, Boulder was a university town of twenty thousand souls snuggled up against the Rocky Mountains—"Five square miles surrounded by reality," as the pundits were fond of saying. Our new home was a place of pink and orange sunsets and semi-arid foothills, a liberal oasis in the middle of a conservative state. There were fitness fanatics and liberal environmentalists and Buddhists and gurus with doctoral degrees waiting tables for a living.

However, most of all, my adopted state was a happy marriage between visible and invisible worlds, with its shortgrass prairies interrupted by a mosaic of farms, its verdant ribbons of cottonwoods, willows, and tamarisk lining sinuous rivers, and higher up there were dense evergreen forests of ponderosa pine and Engleman spruce coating mountain slopes. Golden groves of aspen trees shimmered under autumn's bright sun.

Growing up, I had learned that silence could be dangerous. Silence stretched between two quarreling parents. Silence surrounded the subject of my father's mental illness. Like a nurturing parent providing safe shelter, Colorado helped me break the silence, to bear witness, to make my voice heard. What is intuition but an intent listening to what the universe is saying, the spires of mountains, the stained glass of sun shining through leaves, the *a cappella* choir of water cascading over rocks?

It was in my new home that I learned that silence could also be healing. After a ten-hour shift in Intensive Care, with its high-tech symphony of buzzers and beeps, its wheezing respirators, scared voices, clattering machines, and cream- colored curtains screeching on ball bearings, it was heaven to climb with my small son above timberline into alpine tundra, a fragile ecosystem of grass and flowers and endless winter and pristine silence. Colorado high country taught me that silence could also mean safety and solitude instead of fear and loneliness.

Our Intensive Care Unit consisted of a dozen beds set in small, partitioned, three-sided cubicles along the outside walls of a large room. The fourth side faced the nurses' station, a room within a room. I worked for eight years in the Intensive Care Unit filled with high-pitched voices and clattering metallic equipment and rules. *Three visits a day by family members only. Fifteen minutes a visit.* Tom, a sixty-five-year-old retired engineer, was admitted with end-stage heart disease and was wired to all kinds of machinery and bottles. We hadn't been able to do anything for him. Every day he seemed to take a step backward.

A medical decision needed to be made about how much more medical care Tom wanted. A meeting involving his physician, nurse, wife, and daughter convened by Tom's bed. He looked cadaverous.

"We need to talk about whether you want to be put on a machine if you need help breathing," the cardiologist began. "You can't stay in ICU unless you want everything done, all resuscitative measures."

"I'll have to move?"

"We promise to keep you comfortable," the doctor said.

Tom looked around the large room. Two patients were on respirators. "I wouldn't want to end up like that," he whispered.

Later that day, his doctor made Tom a DNR, Do Not Resuscitate. Comfort was the criterion for his care. "Respond to chest pain with morphine and nitroglycerine. We just want to get him to a medical floor," his doctor instructed. I was the one who transferred Tom to 2 North where he died the next day with his wife and daughter at his bedside.

Just saying the words "hospital nurse" conjured images that could suddenly swirl out of focus: smashed skulls, stapled backs, shaved heads, curved incisions, bandage turbans, surgical drains, crani caps. So many emotions impossible to forget: wincing, whining, tears, giggles, dogged perseverance, confusion, withdrawal, anxiety so strong that it quaked the body sending aftershocks for days. Always it was the sisterhood of nurses that got us through our ten-hour shifts, jumping in to help one another if a patient suddenly took a critical turn. A sisterhood of strong women who knew how to adjust ventilator settings and interpret lab reports, as well as knowing when it was best to be quiet and listen.

Patients arrived at our hospital with hope—ranchers from the Western Slope, a butcher from Telluride, a CEO of a software firm—and I eased them out of their jean jackets and three-piece suits, tied up the backs of their flimsy gowns, and settled them into the ICU environment. Tumors were removed, pain numbed, eyesight saved, walking restored. I have stood in the hall and felt air being sucked out of the room as a surgeon exited, watched as mortality descended on a wife's shoulders, too weak to handle the weight of her husband's illness.

Exhausted after my shift, I returned home to our furnished townhouse with its green shag carpet and the realities of being a single parent: proving that I was a good credit risk, agonizing over finding not only competent, but caring, babysitters. It was all worth it when

I tiptoed in to check on Chris and saw how he had done his usual nocturnal spin, hunched with his rump in the air, his chubby fist poked through the bars of the crib, his half-open mouth, his sweet, low breath.

Voices in the books lining my shelves always called to me. I picked up Emerson and his words sang, "The poet is the only true doctor." Freud whispered, "Everywhere I go I find a poet has been there before me." Flaubert crooned, "One does not choose one's subject matter, one submits to it." And the poet-doctor, William Carlos Williams, who scribbled poems in scattered moments between shooting antibiotics in the rear ends of screaming children, "It is difficult/ to get the news from poems/ yet men die miserably every day/ for lack of what is found there." Even the Bible began with, "In the beginning was the Word."

When I became a graduate student in creative writing at the University of Colorado, I ran from ICU, where I had just taken a chronic lung patient off the respirator, to writing workshops where my fellow students were arguing about the length of term papers. Always I floated on the periphery of the university bubble. All around swirled Black Panther speeches and readings by Allen Ginsberg, founder of the Jack Kerouac School of Disembodied Poetics at Naropa, but there was no extra time for such luxuries.

Poetry 101. There was the usual scuffle as students settled into chairs, their eyes puffy from too little sleep or too abrupt an awakening to attend the ten o'clock class I taught as a teaching assistant.

"Good morning," I said. "Today, I want to discuss how ideas and images come to a writer. Like running, the more you write the better you'll become. Some days you don't feel like running, you're coming down with a cold or have to pay the bills. There will always be interruptions and obstacles. Write whether you want to or not. A poem is never going to emerge on the page perfectly formed. It's hard work. One page leads to two and then, by working every day, you might have something eventually that resembles a book. Just as a runner has to race through cramps and fatigue in order to catch his second wind, you must keep writing through the daydreaming and the list of obligations staring you in the face."

Two women in the front row were taking down every word I said. A young man with dyed black hair, a silver cross dangling from his right ear, and a nose ring sat in the corner. So far he hadn't turned in any assignments.

"Who would like to read the poem I handed out to you last time, 'Pavane for the Passing of a Child, After the music of Ravel' by Laura Chester. Yes, Cindy, go ahead."

"Possible/ that I lift this hand/ feel a weight I've never felt there?/ Possible/ I hold this weight/ collapsed and sunk and tamed now/ feel a flesh so warm gone under/…" Cindy swayed with the rhythm of the words. She read the poem to the end.

"Good. What is the poem about?" I asked.

"Grief. The poet is grieving for her child. I'm not sure if it's because of an accident or an abortion," Cindy said.

"What lines make you think the poem might be about an abortion?"

"The lines 'It sucked and made a vacant space there./ Where there had been a child/ a child no longer./ Collapsed in her./ It sucked her fill.' That seems like an abortion scene," Cindy replied.

"Good."

"I don't see that at all. I think it's just a woman who's lost a child in an accident or maybe to a disease," Alicia said.

"I think the poet is using the loss of a child as a metaphor for any loss."

"We have at least three interpretations about what is going on in this poem," I said. "Does that bother anyone? Should there be one way of interpreting it? Who gave the correct answer?" I waited for someone to have the courage to climb out on that intellectual limb.

"I think it would take the excitement and emotion out of the poem, if you try to analyze each line, be forced to come to one conclusion," Paul, the man with the nose ring, said.

"Yes, that's the wonderful thing about good poetry," I said. You can read it over the breakfast table and get one meaning from it, read it the next day and be enthralled with the rhythm and music in the poet's choice of words, and then read it at midnight and feel the sadness. Good poetry has several layers: the conscious scene with which the poet engages your interest so that you want to read further because you care about what is happening, the personal layer, and then the poem goes beyond to the universal layer that makes the reader say, 'Yes, I understand that. I've been there too.' Poetry is a word collage, placing layer upon layer of images until a poem emerges. Like a visual artist applies layer after layer of oil paint."

"Or like giving birth to a child," Cindy said. "It must feel something like that. There a poem is, a new life that must stand on its own, make its own relationships with other people."

"Good," I replied. "I want you to write for the rest of the period. Write about leaving. Moving to a new town maybe or going through a divorce or what it felt like to leave home to come to college. Don't be abstract. Write details, how the sky looked, what a mess your room was. Focus on honesty and accuracy and details. Just keep your hand moving. Don't edit yourself. Let the images come." For the next fifteen minutes, the only sound was paper being ripped from spiral pads and an occasional cough.

"Good work in class today, Paul," I said, as he slid two pages onto my desk. He smiled and turned red. I watched him leave with Cindy and knew they were discussing the poem about the death of a child.

*　　　*

The voice of the writer may seem to have no more importance than the whining of a cricket in the grass, but creativity lives on by faith even during times of interruption and illness and neglect. Before his lobotomy, my father wrote a one-act play, "Stars Secure." I have a photograph of my father sporting a fake moustache and my mother and another pastor in costume standing near the altar of a church. A newspaper clipping stated that this play was performed several times in front of different congregations. My father wrote poetry and this play, which I've tried, without success, to find. From reading his snatches of poetry and snippets of sermons in the notebook he left behind, my sister's and my only legacy, I imagine that the play was about faith and how it manifests itself in peoples' lives. The tragedy about the lobotomy that my father received in 1947 at Toledo State Hospital was its irreversibility and the destruction of my father's creative imagination.

Poetry makes sense in a way that the high-tech medical procedures I participated in every day as a registered nurse did not. Poetry goes to the essence of things, from the inside out. What science is always trying to take apart, poetry understands and takes in whole. Reading poetry is entering the realm of lilacs and wolves where words sing and ideas dance, a Garden-of-Eden-of-the-Imagination where everything is connected.

Both writers and medical scientists are seekers of truth. However, nothing is real to medical researchers except as an occurrence that happens to a significant number of people, known as "a body of research," whereas nothing is real to a writer except the experience of a single person, which the medical community tends to dismiss as "anecdotal evidence." Truth is more likely to tumble out of a poem than out of an equation, for the poem need not be tested with chemicals or dissection but must only resonate with another soul as true.

The more I studied, the more I realized that writing is like nursing in so many ways. Neither writers nor nurses ever feel that what they have to offer is good enough. Neither are ever done. Close attention must be paid to details or both the poem and the patient will die. Both writers and nurses must keep the faith, persevere, and see the poem or patient through difficult crises. People are the most important ingredient in both professions. You have to be willing to reassess at a moment's notice and embark on another course. Sometimes radical surgery is needed in order for a wound to heal. Telling a story and listening to someone else's is what sacred means. This is what I learned from both of my fathers: the father who gave me life and the father who taught me how to listen, how to live.

⪦ ⪧

Dad Browne suffered a stroke within a month after I moved to Boulder in 1973.

"Should I come?" I asked my mother. Five years earlier my mother and stepfather and two youngest sisters, Kathy and Jeanne, had moved to Toccoa, Georgia, a town of nine thousand whose only claim to fame was a majestic waterfall. When my stepfather retired from his medical practice in Ohio, my mother had chosen Toccoa because there was a Christian high school for my sisters to attend.

"Not necessary," Mother assured me. "The doctors say it was a mild stroke."

A week later she called to tell me that Dad Browne had died. "What happened?"

"He had another more severe stroke," she said. "He wanted to be buried in Whitehouse, to lie next to Kathryn's grave."

"I'll take the next flight to Toledo," I said. I couldn't stop crying. Somehow the grief over the end of my marriage and my stepfather's death became tangled into one huge wound. I shed tears for the death of my biological father and because I had not attended his funeral ten years too late. Grief overtook me like a mugger waiting in a dark alley. I cried during the flight and at the funeral and at night when I couldn't sleep. Looking at the pictures of my stepfather holding my baby son that I had taken on our journey west gave little comfort.

"He stopped taking his blood pressure medication," my sister Barbara told me after the funeral.

"How do you know?" I asked.

"His prescription hadn't been filled for three months," she replied.

What is the truth of a family story? The hard data found in letters and hospital charts and pictures or the emotional truth of how it felt to be carried upstairs in my father's arms? How my stepfather understood me without words and bought me new clothes at a time when I didn't care what I wore? What is love but seeing beauty in another's eyes?

My dear stepfather gave up the fight and committed a more genteel form of suicide—a sin of omission rather than commission. Now my mother relaxed and enjoyed her cottage by Lake Hartwell. She bloomed under her new freedom. I observed all this and couldn't shake the feeling that my mother had driven my stepfather to find a release from their arguments. Within a month of moving to Colorado, I received word that both Grandma and Grandpa Motter had died, too. Having lost their farm to bankruptcy many years before, they had lived in a trailer on my uncle's farm. Grandpa took care of Grandma after she became senile. "He carried her to bed and threw her in and she'd laugh as if he were the greatest comedian who ever lived," a cousin said. A month after she passed on the trailer went up in flames, with my grandfather inside. No one knew if the fire had been an accident or intentional.

⇌ ⇌

The Victorian priest-poet, Gerard Manley Hopkins, coined the word, "inscape," which re-ferred to the way that we human beings can merge with the natural world. For him, inscape was an infinite "map in the head" and "the soul of art." Hopkins wrote, "And for all this, nature is never spent. There lives the dearest precious deep-down things." Every atom, tree, and rock was inscape, a glimpse of universal harmony. Writing in 1870 on the inscape, the strength and grace of a single bluebell, he wrote, "I know the beauty of our Lord by it."

"Instress" was the sensation of "inscape," the word he coined for the stress of God's will in and through all things. He believed that poetry must have moral significance, and the beauty and worth of all things must be seen through the love of God. His poetry was shaped by the tension between the asceticism of his Jesuit faith and the aesthetic values he saw in nature.

Upon entering the Society of Jesus in 1866, Hopkins burned all his poetry and vowed to write no more, a vow he later recanted. His poetry was shaped by his religion, his personal reading of nature, his love of people, and his critical approach to art. The poverty he saw around him in Liverpool, where he worked as a priest, made the melancholia he suffered most of his life more intense. He used creative violence, radical surgery, to break through to a new poetic style using "sprung rhythm." He moved English poetry forward by taking it back to its primal Anglo-Saxon origins by coining and compounding words: "hailropes," "heavengravel," "wanwood." A distant hill became "a slow tune."

On days off from my job in Intensive Care, I drove into the mountains near our home. I carried my son onto the Upper Burning Bear Creek Trail, and before us lay a high-coun-try collage of clear tumbling water and meadows yawning below. We climbed up into thick forest, a green mansion, an ancient cathedral. Mighty columns soared to the vault where boughs intertwined like hands clasped in prayer. Slender beams of amber sunlight flickered, as if in medieval dimness. Pine needles were incense. Birds and bats fluttered within their niches. In this hush, I waited for an unseen organ to crash into "Te Deum."

As we rounded a curve in the trail, there before us was a soaring spine of mountains. Sunlight made a purple halo against blue sky and large clouds and the sway of trees. We crossed a footbridge over Burning Bear Creek as it whispered its way through a twisted course of oxbows and meanders. We stopped on the footbridge and listened to the creek water calling below. I bent down to look more closely and saw insect larvae, with their disc-shaped suction cups at the rear of their bodies like tiny anchors chaining them to the slippery surface of stones. A caddis fly wove a small net, floated into the stream in an attempt to trap morsels of food. A silvery glint of trout streaked through water, slalomed around rocks. Frogs chanted "jug-o-rum, jug-o-rum." Solitude was a great antidote to the loud machines in Intensive Care—the sweet perfume of starflowers and chickenweed and chokeberry.

Like Hopkins, when I want to feel God I return to the mountains and forest, cathedral-like with its coolness and dim light and silence. The outer path leads inward past great buttresses of giant pines interspersed with straight white columns of aspen. Awe and exultation come easily standing in a forest, but there's also the feeling that it's all too vast, too impersonal, too deeply shadowed, and my life is truly insignificant. All sounds, an inexplicable gurgle or a whistle, gain enhanced mystery as I blend into the landscape.

Grand Lake is a mirror reflecting spired evergreens and lodgepole pines, all the golds and umbers and coppers of a Rocky Mountain autumn. A spider does his spider-paddle across water, climbs out on shore, and wobbles away. Beneath the lake's silvery ceiling there is a whole other world of prowlers and spinners and burrowers.

Mountains grow and pulsate and decay. Stones possess power. In order to see the greatness of a mountain, it is necessary to keep a distance. To understand its form, you must move around it; in order to experience its moods, you must observe it at sunrise and sunset, at noon and midnight, in sun and in rain. With wails and roars and trills, wind rushes through branches and apertures, like breath, then is still. The incense of pine needles and wet jeans rise around me.

Humus means "fertile soil" and is the root word for "humility." With another suffix, the word becomes "human." Did the Earth become human or did humans emerge from the Earth? Answers lie in cognates such as "humble" and "humane," which extend the meaning of both Earth and ourselves. The word "wiros" is the first root for man, which takes on a vain connotation in the words "virile" and "virtue," but also turns into the Germanic word "weraldh," meaning the life of man, and from there, into our English "world." Etymology tells us the world of man is derived from this planet, shares origins with the life of the soil, and if it wants to survive, must learn to live in humility with the rest of life. If only we learn that lesson before it is too late.

The overhead light created a tableau as a young woman stood by her father's bed, tears rolling down her cheeks. John lay in our ICU, comatose after suffering a stroke, with the respirator breathing for him and intravenous medications maintaining his heart rate and blood pressure. "When will he wake up? When will he be able to breathe without the machine?" John's wife and daughter asked me, and of course I couldn't give them an answer. He reminded me of my stepfather who had died of a stroke several years before. People trust the medical community to help them. Sometimes we can't. Sometimes high-tech makes things worse, leaving the patient with no way out. If John hadn't been resuscitated and placed on life-support, he would have died naturally when the stroke happened.

Later that afternoon, Dr. Grayson arrived. We went into John's room for a family conference. The only sound was the rhythmic whooshing of the respirator. Dr. Grayson nodded at me. I touched John's arm. No movement. I watched air being pushed through his breathing tube. His chest rose and fell, rose and fell, in slow, regular movements. I disconnected the alarm on the monitor. With one hand, I disconnected the breathing tube, and with the other, I stroked John's arm. Hearing is the last sense to go.

"I'm disconnecting the breathing tube, John. You won't feel pain. Soon your suffering will be over," I said.

"We're here with you, John," his wife said. The printout of his heart rate fell sharply and then stopped. I removed the equipment and positioned him so that he looked comfortable. His wife and daughter stayed for another hour. Death can be a compassionate act.

Medicine's approach to health is based upon the perception that healing power is external, chemotherapy or radiation for instance, instead of from the inscape of soul, the ability of the body to rally when faced with life-threatening illness. The philosopher Arthur Schopenhauer said that the only God discernible in nature is the will to live. The body is an instrument of the soul that sometimes plays the blues, sometimes sings hymns, but always the body hums along. Chemicals can't ease the pain of a suffering soul. Health is a matter of the heart, of what we take in or eliminate in our lives, a journey toward balance, connectedness, meaning, and wholeness.

Longing is your teacher. Keep feeding your desires. Say yes instead of no. Voice is the body given away in the world, the whisper of lovers in the night as they make their inner and outer worlds one. Body language is the inscape of music bubbling through alveoli, a poem of synapses firing in the brain, body as vessel for sound and feeling. God, like love, is a verb rather than a noun. God is the "Great I Am," active, always in motion, an ocean of being, the sun rising each morning. Salvation is seeing snow dust the top of mountains.

Chapter Nine

⌒ ARE YOU OKAY? YES, I'M OKAY. ⌒

July sun was tenacious, a hot, muggy day in South Carolina. The concrete parking lot reflected sunlight and heat as my cab came to its final stop in front of Hilton Head Hospital. The sight of the building looming over the trees always brought ambivalent feelings of hope and fear. The puncturing of flesh never fails to startle, just as the invasion of plastic tubes and steel needles never fails to leave my mind quivering. Pain is exhausting simply because I never get used to it.

First stop was Admissions, then up the elevator to my room. It was 1991 and treatment number five. Middle of July, midday heat, halfway through the scheduled immunomodulatory treatments. As usual, I signed a document making sure I knew that Medenica Clinic was a research facility and that I was being given treatment, the efficacy of which had yet to be proven.

I was here because of one moment in 1983 when I was given the Heptavax-B vaccine by my employer. No one told me about the vaccine's risks. I never questioned the vaccine's safety. My son was eleven, and I had been a single parent for nine and a half years. "Be part of the solution instead of part of the problem," my mother had always told me, so when I became an evening supervisor of the hospital where I had worked for eight years, I hoped to make a difference. I listened as nurses told me that they wanted flextime and a nursery in the hospital for their children and grants for continuing education. When a new director of nursing wanted to make the staff all registered nurses, I grieved along with my co-workers as licensed practical nurses were let go amid a storm of protests and tears. The nursing director explained that it was not part of my job to conduct meetings where nurses could air their complaints.

"You are part of the administration now," she said.

"Aren't hospitals here to help nurses help patients?" I asked.

All around me, nurses became silent. "I'm afraid I'll lose my job if I complain," they said.

Two years earlier, I had earned my graduate degree in creative writing after many nights of coming home from work and writing long into the night. Life was busy but rewarding. Summer heat was receding into one of the most beautiful Colorado autumns in memory when I received the second dose of the Heptavax-B vaccine, a sting of needle under skin, one moment that forever changed my life.

Aspens in the foothills near my home had their brightness knobs turned up to their highest levels; the view from my window was a mosaic of stained glass reds, oranges, yellows, and browns. October 28, 1983. After a night of intense pain and fever, I called in sick and pulled sheets up over my shaking body. The shift the night before was the last one I would ever work as a registered nurse.

⌇ ⌇

Now I was on Hilton Head Island, the resort where the Clintons trekked for their Renaissance Weekend, their elitist, wonkish, schmooze immortalized in *The New York Times* as "the saturnalia of soul-searching by the sea," an island of expensive hotels and gourmet restaurants. That this was where my hope for medical treatment resided was the most sadistic of ironies. Once again, I knew that God had a strange sense of humor.

I had replayed this scenario many times in the eight years since my illness began; I sat in a doctor's office, nervously waiting for him to probe various parts of my body and history not generally open to public scrutiny. As I sat on the exam table, my worry filled the small room, air heavy with awareness that decisions would be made by yet another doctor, usually male, his white coat starched with authority. I agreed to reveal my age, weight, current medications, past and present symptoms, stripped myself of reticence along with my slacks and sweater, and answered his questions as part of an implicit agreement: *Patient tells all; doctor cures all.* Tomorrow would be the day my team of doctors would have the answers. What had begun as innocently as a lingering flu had exploded into a full-blown mystery disease, the ever-changing blue in a kaleidoscope through which the rest of my life must be viewed.

This was immunomodulatory therapy number five in a series of ten treatments for systemic lupus erythematosus, systemic vasculitis. Eight years worth of cycling through prednisone and cytoxin and anti-malarial medications as well as more traditional treatments for lupus back home in Colorado had not improved my physical condition. I was having lunch with a friend when, all of a sudden, I couldn't speak. I don't know how she got me to her car. My "transient ischemic attack," the first act before a stroke finale, was what made my doctors decide that my best hope for remaining alive were immunomodulatory treatments, which consisted of large doses of interferon and solumedrol and having my blood cleansed by a plasmapheresis machine.

The immunologist who was treating me in Hilton Head was from Yugoslavia and resembled an exhausted lounge act more than a high-profile physician. Dr. Medenica wore a red plaid sport jacket and a white shirt unbuttoned at the collar. His nose was long and curved, and although his body fit his tall frame proportionately, his face was jowly. He was going bald, and his hair ringed his head like a monk's. His words were wrapped in a heavy Slavic accent. If a movie were made of his life, Karl Malden would star.

I waited in a small room to get blood drawn and to give a urine sample. The young lab technician applied a rubber tourniquet and missed my vein twice. "Try this arm," I suggested, noting the sweat gathering on his forehead. Three was a charmed number. Dark vermilion flowed up the tube, and my arm received its badge of honor. Urine, unlike blood, was bountiful. On to the EKG lab. Then it was time for what I dreaded most, the insertion of the subclavian catheter. Every month, I closed my eyes, tried to relax, and took a few slow, rhythmic breaths as I felt pressure under my clavicle and then a pop as the catheter was threaded up my subclavian vein. The portable chest X-ray checked to make sure the catheter wasn't lodged in my lung by mistake.

"We're ready for you, Connie," Patti said, as she smoothed her blue scrubs with her small hands. "What's your musical taste today?"

"Enya," I said. Patti helped me pass the four hours I was hooked up to the plasmapheresis machine by telling jokes. Laughter, an analgesic releasing endorphins more potent than morphine. Laughter, the best antidote to machines. But the treatments were no joke. It was a strange feeling to watch my blood circling outside my body through plastic coils, mine but not mine. From all the years I worked as a registered nurse, I remembered how fresh blood, ripped from body parts, smelled, an aroma that went straight to some deep primitive center of the cortex. Once the subclavian catheter was in place, the procedure was painless, but always there was the nagging worry in the back of my mind: *Do this nurse and this technician know what they're doing?* My apprehension was not exactly allayed by the fact that there was a high turnover in staffing at the clinic. It was difficult for hospital workers to find housing on this expensive resort island.

"I've got a good joke for you, Connie," Patti said, as she settled in next to my bed. Carefully she gauged the speed with which blood left my body and passed through the machine that separated my red blood cells and plasma and scrubbed it clean of antigens, the foreign substances that caused my autoimmune illness—lupus erythematosus.

"A woman went into an expensive restaurant and asked the busy waiter for a Hilton Head turkey. 'Yes, ma'am, I'll bring it right out,' he said. He went into the kitchen and told the chef a lady had ordered a Hilton Head turkey. The waiter brought the order out on a platter. The woman took the lid off the platter, looked at the bird, and stuck two fingers in its rear end. 'No, no, take it back. This is not a Hilton Head turkey!' she exclaimed.

"'Oh, I'm sorry, ma'am, I'll bring one right away.' He hurriedly brought the platter back to the kitchen and said, 'Gee, Chef, this woman really knows her birds. She only wants a Hilton Head turkey.'

"'Okay, that's what she'll get,' the chef muttered. The waiter brought it into the woman and set the platter in front of her. She took off the lid and inserted two fingers in the rear end of the bird.

"'Ah yes,' she said. 'Now THIS is a Hilton Head turkey.'

"'Good, I'm glad to hear it,' the relieved waiter said.

"'You have an accent, where are you from?' the woman asked.

"'Why don't YOU tell me,' the waiter said, as he turned away and bent over."

We finished laughing, and Patti switched my IV bottles. Eyes closed, I concentrated on listening to Enya and imagining sitting by Grand Lake, my favorite place in the world. I was having a picnic with Chris, as our dogs, Brittainy and Bambi, took turns chasing the ball. I imagined that a million filters were siphoning off the immune complexes that clogged my veins. I was sinking down into lake water only to rise reborn. I was kissing a lover I had not yet met.

"Dr. Medenica wants to try this new medication, Gamma-Gard," Patti said, as she hung a new bottle. Within minutes, I felt my trachea closing off. "Patti, help me," I whispered, as I sat straight up in bed and yanked off the earphones. All of my fight-or-flight responses kicked in, my sympathetic nervous system firing away like marines responding to attack. Stasis, that moment of holding air in, absolute standstill, then my neck felt like it was taking on the shape of a blowfish. Patti took one look at me and turned off the medicine and stuck an oxygen cannula in my nose.

"Call Medenica," Patti yelled to the tech in the next room.

"So that's what a drug reaction feels like," I whispered. "I never knew they were so scary."

"Don't let anyone give you Gamma-Gard again," she said.

"No kidding," I replied. My breathing returned to normal. Dr. Medenica arrived and listened to my chest while Patti described my reaction. My life depended on the skill of this nurse. One miscalculation, one oversight, and it would all be over. Assessment skills were the unique, singular skill of a registered nurse, the vigilant mother at the bedside. The physician was the absent father. Sometimes just being able to breathe is a poem.

⌒ ⌒

According to an ancient Egyptian creation story, the creator's first act was to pluck a reed, split its tip, and write the world into existence. The Australian aborigines described the creator as first emerging from the formless void and singing the world into existence—words put to music. Words, the smallest unit of language, translated into objects, feelings, memories, fantasies. The treeness of trees. Middle C on a violin. A sleeping dog. Bestowing names gave power, word magic.

Diagnosis, part of medicine's love for big words and ritual, was necessary in order to prescribe treatment for my illness and hopefully to provide a cure. Early in 1984, I was thrown into a game of diagnostic roulette. *Isolate the symptom. Devise a compensation mechanism for all the life changes.* After a year of diagnostic procedures, I still wandered in an alien land of semantics. Nothing definitive to report. No malignancy. No chromosomal abnormality. As new symptoms arose—blood in urine, high blood pressure, pain in arms and legs, intermittent fever, rashes, run-over-by-a-truck fatigue—my doctor sent me to see an oncologist, a rheumatologist, a nephrologist, more than twelve specialists in all. My lymph nodes were biopsied, then my arteries, and then a lump in my breast. All of them confirmed that my symptoms were real, but no one was able to attach a diagnosis to my constellation of complaints. An open kidney biopsy, done in January 1984, revealed "proliferative glomerulopathy, diffuse, generalized."

"I think you have polyarteritis nodosa," my nephrologist said. "Medical literature is full of hepatitis B as the cause of polyarteritis nodosa and other diseases of the blood vessels. Have you ever had hepatitis B?"

"No," I replied. "But I did receive the hepatitis B vaccine." That information seemed irrelevant to him. I became used to hearing, "This is not the usual clinical picture. Could be lymphoma or lupus erythematosus or henoch-schonlein purpura." Not your everyday, garden variety, movie-of-the-week type of diagnoses.

Three-forty a.m. I was wide awake because of a new roommate. It was the winter of 1984 and my fourth day at Presbyterian Hospital in Denver. The old lady in the next bed rattled the side rails, her mouth pulled up like a purse string, with only a faint whistle escaping. From the look of her, she was not long for this world, but she kept trying to rise to the surface, only to slide once again down to a murky level.

The next morning, I was scheduled for a muscle biopsy and other tests and then planned to be discharged. When I returned to my room in mid-afternoon, the bed next to mine was vacant and held fresh linen. The nurse who helped me into bed also held out a paper for me to sign.

"What's this?" I asked but already knew what she wanted me to sign. "Orders for Resuscitative Measures."

"We need to know what you want done if...it's standard procedure...we ask all patients to sign one," she stammered. I knew all too well what being resuscitated meant. How many times, in the twenty years I worked as a registered nurse, had I brought pink back to skin that had been gray? Intubation. Cardioversion. Vasopressors. Anti-arrhythmic drugs. Defibrillation. And if all else failed, there was always a pacemaker and a respirator.

When it became clear to my employer that I wouldn't be able to return to my nursing supervisor position, I received letters from the Director of Nursing that it was incumbent upon me to apply for Social Security Disability. In March 1984, I was proclaimed "totally physically disabled" by my doctors but still didn't have a definitive medical diagnosis. Meanwhile, the world trundled on. The Mets won the World Series. Gorbachev cleaned out the Kremlin. The Berlin Wall came tumbling down. Neighbors and friends got dressed every morning and left for work or class, and I made the rounds of oncologist, rheumatologist, and nephrologist.

Being a patient meant being awakened at four in the morning for blood pressure checks, hanging modesty up in the closet along with my jeans, and being palpated and poked with needles. Being a patient meant lab techs and nurses paraded through my room on their schedule instead of mine. Being a patient was praying for divine compassion but never knowing if God was listening. Being a patient was a fast freefall in the dark, the shock of impermanence, the panic of not knowing where the bottom lay.

I, like all nurses, suffered from denial, a belief that illness could not happen to me. My generation of nurses had grown up with antibiotics and vaccines and blind faith that most diseases could be treated. "Science has made modern medicine safe," was the covert lesson I was taught in nurse's training, along with the muscles of the hand. Safety was an agreed upon myth; otherwise, who would fill the nursing trenches? During my two decades in the field, I saw how nurses had become the unhappy spouses in their marriage to medicine. The marriage wasn't working, but no one knew what to do to make it better. Patients were the latchkey children of this volatile union, the innocents who often experienced the inadequacy of the health care safety net.

I began a second career as a medical sleuth, reading textbooks about vaccines—the holy grail, the consummate wafer of disease prevention. Vaccines were made from bacteria or viruses and were in either live or killed preparations. Live viruses were attenuated, or weakened, by using one of several methods such as filtering a virus strain through animal cells fifty or more times to reduce potency. A second form of immunization was done with killed vaccines in which the organisms were inactivated by the use of radiation, heat, or chemicals. The Heptavax-B vaccine, which I received in 1983, was of the killed-preparation variety. The vaccine, laden with formaldehyde and ethylmercury (thimerosal) used as preservatives, was a twentieth century version of Macbeth's witches' brew: "eye of newt and toe of frog."

As I lay at home on the couch, the air was the bronze-gold of a Rembrandt landscape. Red and brown leaves peeked out from behind green cottonwoods. Yellow jackets looped, while ants scurried up and down the sidewalk, bearing their sweet burden. Chuang Tzu, who helped craft the tenets of Taoism in ancient China over two millennia ago, suggested that the most profound forms of communication go beyond words. He wrote, "Words exist because of meaning; once you've got the meaning, you can forget the words." Once again solitude became my comforting partner.

"Come with me to Louisville. I want to look at an antique lamp," I had said to my ten-year-old son two years before everything changed. We had moved to a home near Boulder that I had bought the year I became supervisor at the hospital.

"Do I have to?" Chris didn't share my enthusiasm for antiques. We had no furniture when we arrived in Boulder in 1973 and had lived in a furnished apartment until I gradually was able to buy furniture. Slowly over the years, I had furnished our home with walnut antiques— a walnut table, six chairs, a walnut secretary, and several bookcases to hold my growing library. The love of old wood and the stories that antiques told were a legacy from my stepfather.

I stopped the car in front of a house in Louisville. There was a sign on the lawn, "Golden Retriever puppies for sale." Chris looked at the sign, his eyes growing huge, and then he looked at me. "Merry Christmas, sweetheart. You can pick out your puppy." From the litter of ten pups, one of them gamboled into my son's arms and into our hearts.

"This is the best Christmas ever, Mom," Chris said, as he played with Brittainy under the Christmas tree. Brittainy was Chris' companion and bed partner. Her cold nose had kissed him good night. Her teeth had chewed everything in sight, including transforming poplar saplings at the back of our yard into nubbins.

Now, two years later, there was no excuse for my negligence. I had been at home between hospitalizations when it became clear that Brittainy was going to become a mother. Having her spayed had been on my "to-do" list, but buying Chris a winter coat had to be my priority. Brittainy's pregnancy was the result of a one-night stand with our neighbor's dashing black Labrador-Great Dane mix who, in a fit of passion, had leapt over our fence as if it were invisible. Animals' motivations are so pure—no phone calls not returned, no coquettish glances. He wanted her, she wanted him. So simple. Unfortunately, there was no "morning-after" pill for dogs.

Brittainy's labor began around noon on a Saturday. Chris watched anxiously while Brittainy panted and produced her offspring, which turned into a long process. One brown head appeared. An hour later, a slimy second. A half-hour later, one tiny black bullet-head, confirming paternity as clearly as any blood test.

"Time for bed, Chris," I yelled from the top of the stairs.

"Let me sleep here tonight." Brittainy's head lay in Chris' lap as she panted. "I'll get my sleeping bag."

"Will you be all right?"

"Sure," he said, as he snuggled down.

In the morning, there were two more brown puppies and one more black one, seven in all. Chris was the proud, sleep-deprived papa. Brittainy was trying to catch a nap with a pup pulling at each nipple. It was late afternoon when I persuaded Chris that he should go out to play. "Brittainy needs her rest," I said, gently guiding him up the stairs.

When we checked on our nursery the next morning, two of the brown puppies were dead. Brittainy took turns licking one, then the other, as if trying to awaken them. Chris started to cry, "I shouldn't have left her." And I whipped myself for not taking Brittainy to the vet when her labor dragged on. Maybe I should have moved the pups to another area; maybe Brittainy accidentally smothered them.

It was immediately clear that Brittainy was grieving. Whenever I tried to remove the two dead puppies, she bared her teeth. She had never so much as growled at me before. I watched as she nuzzled her dead pups, dangled her nipples near their still mouths, as if coaxing them to take hold.

The next day, Chris and I buried the pups in the backyard and held a funeral. I recited "The Lord's Prayer" while Chris wiped away tears. My son learned about birth and death all in the same weekend.

"Are you going to die, too, Mama?" he asked, pain in his voice because grief was still a strange language. "Every time you go into the hospital, I wonder if you'll come home."

"The doctors have to do a lot of tests so they know what kind of medicine to give me," I said. "Don't worry, I'm very stubborn. I'm going to be around a long, long time."

As always when I needed guidance, I turned to the poets for truth. The poet Rainier Maria Rilke's answer to uncertainty was, "Be patient toward all that is unsolved in your heart, and try to love the questions themselves, like locked rooms and like books that are written in a very foreign tongue. Do not seek the answers, which cannot be given you, because you would not be able to live them. Live the questions now. Perhaps you will then gradually, without noticing it, live along some distant day into the answer."

Fall 1986. I was ushered into the exam room at National Jewish Hospital in Denver, a cubicle as monochromatic and windowless as a jail cell. The young immunologist examined me calmly, as if I were his only patient all afternoon. The thick chart that my primary physician had sent him lay open on the desk.

"I think you have a vasculitic condition caused by the Heptavax-B vaccine you received back in 1983," the immunologist said slowly. "I've been treating a man who has experienced a similar chronology of events."

"I've wondered about that, because I became so ill within two days of the second dose," I said.

"That's when hypersensitivity symptoms often occur," he replied. "It's like a serum sickness that refuses to go away."

"What kind of treatment do you recommend?" I was on the edge of my seat in anticipation of ending this nightmare of disability.

"Your doctors have already tried prednisone, anti-malarial drugs, and cytoxin. There's one other thing we can do if you get worse," he said. "Plasmapheresis, but I hope that won't be necessary. All we can do is treat symptoms as they arise," he said, as he took my hand, a gesture of sympathy. Symptoms, the language the body speaks when under fire, can be a source of valuable information or a prison sentence. After eight years of total disability, I finally received a diagnosis: "systemic lupus erythematosus, systemic vasculitis, glomerulonephritis induced by the hepatitis vaccine." My body was constantly fighting the foreign substance introduced by the vaccine. Like the Trojan horse, the enemy was inside. Lupus strikes patients when they are in the prime of life, 90 percent of whom are women.

The mystic Julian of Norwich wrote that severe illness brought on "revelations, the wondrous appearance of the Lord Himself." She said that pain produced contradictory responses, "fury at the force that was a disturbing distraction and at another time the rare opportunity to see everything more vividly, with a clarity I could only wonder at, in which the details of my present life were intensified and acutely delineated. Pain is a form of information, a language all its own."

Dr. Shiovitz washed his hands after examining me. "I was hoping that the prednisone and cytoxin would help you feel better. So far it doesn't seem to be making much difference, but I've been a doctor long enough to know that malignant tumors can mysteriously disappear. So-called incurable patients recover, and we doctors, if we're honest, credit it to an act of God. Or, if we're not honest, we claim that we had the magical cure. All any of us can really do is to accept health with a bewildered sense of gratitude."

"It would be easy to go to bed and stay there," I said.

"I'm a firm believer in the power of old-fashioned anger working through each one of us," my doctor said. "Martin Luther King would never have started the Civil Rights Movement if he hadn't gotten really angry about not being served at a lunch counter. Van Gogh wouldn't have painted his masterpieces if he hadn't failed as a minister of the Gospel among the coal miners."

"I'm going to do some research to see if there's any link between vaccines and chronic illnesses," I said.

"I'd be interested in reading what you find. I'll see you through this," he replied.

Anger gave me the energy to roll out of bed in the morning, to get my son off to school, to work at my word processor. Anger gave me the energy to spend many hours researching medical journal articles, documenting side effects and long-term disabilities caused by vaccines. Anger was the life force that helped me submit a Freedom of Information request to the Food and Drug Administration about any research linking Heptavax-B vaccine to chronic illnesses. Six months later, I received a printout that said there were seven other documented cases of systemic vasculitis following inoculation with Heptavax-B vaccine. No names, only numbers. Nine months later, a huge carton arrived in the mail, containing computer printouts from the Vaccine Adverse Reporting System (VAERS). With a sinking heart, I read all the vascular problems listed—heart attacks, strokes, perforated bowels—as well as more mild symptoms such as rashes, muscular pain, and fever.

"Number 333383: A fifty-eight-year-old male physician who developed myalgia, arthralgia, fatigue, serous otitis media, transient loss of vision in one eye and multiple peripheral neuropathies following the third injection of Heptavax-B. He is currently being treated with cytoxin and prednisone for a polyarterititis-like illness."

In response to a letter I wrote to the manufacturer of the vaccine, I received the following response: "Your letter of inquiry dated May 16, 1988 concerning Heptavax-B has been forwarded to my attention. Since Heptavax-B has been on the market, we have received occasional reports of vasculitis following vaccinations. We would be interested in receiving additional information concerning any patient you may be treating who has such a diagnosis."

My first introduction to the dark side of medicine had been many years before, when I researched my father's lobotomy, trying to find out why that surgery had been permitted to continue for so many years. Now I was once again face-to-face with medical intrigue—cloak-and-dagger discovery of new drugs. One health maintenance organization stealing patients from another. The political intrigue of American Medical Association lobbyists. The duel for international prestige. The race to cure AIDS or cancer or Alzheimer's. Dumping mental patients in the next county or state so someone else's taxes will pick up the tab.

Back in 1983, no clinical trials of new drugs were done on women before they were approved by the FDA. "They are too difficult and expensive to study," the pharmaceutical companies said. They even tested estrogen therapy on men, even used male rats. Men's bodies have always been taken as the norm. It was also men who were the CEOs of the major pharmaceutical companies and the chief immunologists of university research departments who were paid by the pharmaceutical companies to do clinical trials. Men were the paid medical experts who presented the clinical trials to the Food and Drug Administration for their approval. *Danger, warning, at risk* were the red flags the health care behemoth waved to keep troops moving in lockstep. *Right, left, right, left.* And there I stood in line like a good soldier, my arm bared for the bullet.

⇒ ⇐

Three a.m. often found me awake with only my fellow travelers in the land of insomnia to keep me company. "Sleep," Vladimir Nabokov wrote, "is the most moronic fraternity in the world, with the heaviest dues and crudest rituals." The diaries of Franz Kafka were full of entries such as, "Slept. Awoke. Slept. Awoke. Miserable life. Let me only have rest at night— childish complaint," which attested to his lifelong battle with insomnia. Thomas Alva Edison, a strong-willed, high-energy person, tried to sleep only four or five hours a night so that he would have time to work on his creative projects. "Most people overeat 100% and oversleep 100%... That extra 100% makes them unhealthy and inefficient." Edison hoped that his lightbulb would help people trim off that excess 100 percent. Swedish film director, Ingmar Bergman, said, "For the past fourteen years I can barely manage four hours sleep a night. I've succeeded in exorcising my insomnia thanks to books and music. I'd imagine that Tolstoy and Mozart, among others, have literally saved my life."

It was usually money worries that kept me wide awake. My every humiliation and shortcoming paraded around in my brain. Disability pay was not enough to cover our bills. When I saw an ad in the paper that a meditation group wanted to rent a room for five hours a week, I called, and a very kind voice was on the other end of the phone.

One night a month later, my writing group was sitting around my table, sharing poetry and tea and laughter, when a loud "Ommmm" levitated up the basement stairs.

"What was that?" Marcia asked.

"Just some people in my basement," I said, turning red.

"Connie has a church in her basement," Morgan laughed.

"Could be worse things," Sarah said.

The Self-Realization Fellowship, with their pictures of Mahatma Gandhi and Martin Luther King and Jesus, brought much needed income and gentle karma to my small home.

Over the next nine years, there were two women who rented one of our bedrooms so that I could pay the mortgage. "Are you okay with this, Chris?" I asked. He was entering his teens, and I knew how he loved his privacy. He worked after school in a supermarket in order to have money for clothes and for movies with his friends.

"If it means keeping the house, let's do it," he said.

Marjorie was soft-spoken and wafer thin and a graduate of Naropa, the local Buddhist college. She had been born with a cleft lip, which gave her mouth a perpetual sneer, which she compensated for by smiling a lot. She had a degree in psychology and furnished her room with a futon and a schefflera and a lamp that gave off a pink glow.

"Stagnant energy causes illness," she said, when I told her that I had lupus. "Let me open your chakras." I had tried acupuncture and Chinese herbs, so why not open my chakras?

Life with Marjorie in the house was peaceful; we shared books and often meals. Three months into our landlord-tenant-budding-friendship relationship, Marjorie shared one of her dreams with me.

"My breast is crying," she said. She showed me a drawing of her breast with dark shadows.

"Does your breast hurt?" I asked.

"I have a sore," she said, as if she were talking about a rainstorm.

"Do you want to show me? I used to be a nurse," I replied.

When she took off her blouse and bra, a piece of gauze covered a weeping hole in her right breast. *Cancer,* my mind cried. "How long has it looked like this?"

"Maybe three months," she said

"Do you have a doctor?" I asked.

"No. I've been doing visualizations and prayer," she replied.

"Will you see my doctor? I think this is serious," I pleaded.

I drove her to my doctor's office and from there to a surgeon's office, who scheduled Marjorie for a biopsy the next day. A few days later, she told me the biopsy showed cancer.

"What are you going to do? Have a mastectomy? Chemo?" I asked.

"I'm going to continue with what I've been doing, visualizations and prayer," Marjorie said. Nothing I said could persuade her otherwise. She was self-employed and had no health insurance. Money was a big part of her decision, but what I saw in her was resignation at her fate rather than peaceful acceptance. She had given in, given up, been beaten down long before she moved into my home. I wanted to give her a transfusion of anger and problem-solving and determination to fight for her life. Unfortunately, the will to live must be a self-transfusion, like the new machines that recycle spilled blood and give it back to its owner. She stayed two more months and then moved in with a friend. A year later, I read her obituary in the newspaper.

If I wasn't a nurse anymore, who was I? My illness made me speak out in a way that I never had before. The worst had happened. What did I have to lose? In her essay, "On Being Ill," Virginia Woolf spoke of the sense of freedom illness conferred. She wrote, "There is, let us confess, a childish outspokenness in illness, things are said, trusts blurted out, which the cautious respectability of health conceals…With responsibility shelved and reason in abeyance—for who is going to exact criticism from an invalid or sound sense from the bedridden?—other tastes assert themselves; sudden, fitful, intense."

Buddhists maintain that illness is an opportunity for enlightenment, for burning off negative karma. Because illness is so intensely personal, there are truths as different as each person's eye color or DNA or dreams. "Why has this happened to me?" is the universal question of the ill. Like a pile of leaves on a forest floor, bodies break down, fall apart. Termites, ticks, fungi, viruses, agents of decay are always at work in the timberline forest of the body. Hippocrates, the Father of Medicine, said illness was cured by "coction" or boiling. One of the Navajo words for disease translates as "fragmentation and reassemblage." Medicine keeps stumbling along in search of a new paradigm, a golden mean that can somehow bridge the Cartesian split between mental and physical worlds.

≈   ≈

All of a sudden, my son was a six-foot-four, sixteen-year-old high school student and embarrassed if I hugged him in public. Nervously, I went through the mother-son rite of passage of teaching Chris how to drive. We spent hours in the car together, while I urged him to please let his foot off the gas and to please use the turn signal.

"Remember to breathe," I said, a reminder to myself as well. Sometimes when I looked at my six-foot-four son, I still saw the little boy who had sobbed over a burst balloon, a large red one he had received on his fourth birthday. The six-year-old who had learned how to ride his bike as I ran alongside, steadying his ride with my hand. The trick was knowing when to let go.

Chris hummed while he made popcorn in the microwave, a mindless tune, the melody unrecognizable, a musical cul-de-sac going nowhere. His hum was more a reflex action, like talking in his sleep. He wasn't aware of it. I loved it because it was a barefoot-in-the-grass, sneaking-out-the-back-door kind of hum. Not like my hum, full of worry about biopsy reports and medical treatments and paying the mortgage. Chris was at the age when the only medicine he needed was prunes and nothing was more exciting than a basketball game or phone call from a friend.

His hum brought memories of his pockets full of rocks and bottle caps and mischief. A shoe box with airholes that served as a hospital for an injured grasshopper. Dirty knees and dirty hands and long legs covered with scabs. Sometimes he slipped up and called me Mama, but mostly he thought he was too old for that. The day he got his driver's license, he gave me a hug, and he blew me a kiss from across the street before he went for his first drive alone.

≈   ≈

Armed with what I believed was irrefutable evidence of a link between my illness and the Heptavax-B vaccine, I decided to pursue a workers' compensation claim. If a play were written about vaccine-related illness, the three acts would be: Act I: *This couldn't happen, a nurse becoming ill from a vaccine that was supposed to protect her.* Act II: *The threat of shunning, if she dared break silence.* Act III: *Speaking out and letting the chips fall where they may.*

"Just calling to wish you luck," Pat said. "Dave and I are praying for you."

"I'm just going to speak the truth," I said. "The letters from my doctors should be all that I need to prove what happened. But Dr. Shiovitz thought they might bring up our father's mental hospital incarceration, so he had me see a psychologist to be tested."

"After all this time?" she asked. "That's terrible."

"No, he was just trying to cover all the arguments they might bring up," I replied. "The psychologist said I'm coping with the illness well. How many people can say they have a medical document proving they're not crazy!"

"I could have told them that," she said.

"If I haven't gone crazy by now, I never will, dear sister. I love you."

The day of my workers' compensation hearing, June 28, 1991, was so hot that tiny black bubbles of tar ballooned on the parking lot. I stepped through the heavy doors of the court-house into total blackness. Concentric rows of seats and shiny oak rails and the judge's bench gradually came into focus. Everything was on the line with this lawsuit: financial solvency, personal integrity, and continued health care. I had letters from three of my physicians stat-ing their belief that my illness was caused by the Heptavax-B vaccine I had received while working as a registered nurse. My medical records were a six-inch high tome. Not a best-seller or an easy read. More a mystery than a romance novel.

As I sat in the shelter of my lawyer's large frame, I listened and prayed. Back and forth, arguments and accusations flew. The hearing hopped from minutiae ("Which lot number was the vaccine from?") to the big picture ("That vaccine Ms. Studer received was pulled off the market in 1986"). As my lawyer, my town crier, my Socrates spoke up for my rights, I understood that American jurisprudence was mastering millions of rules and then ap-plying them. Competing value systems. Strategies of legal argument. Persuasion. Nothing could be taken for granted. Nothing was proven just because it was strongly felt. The judge would not be swayed by an emotional declaration of faith. I was awarded back pay, as well as a monthly stipend and health care coverage. Naive woman that I am, I thought I was all done with hearings and judges, but there were many more to come.

Throughout the six years of hearings, one question reverberated in my brain: "*Who are these people?*" Did the Colorado Compensation Authority deliberately recruit their policy-makers and naysayers of treatment from a small subset of Americans who had no experi-ence with illness? Having to prove my injuries over and over to a group of bureaucrats, in spite of my physicians' documentation, felt like further injury. Winning my workers' com-pensation suit was a sobering joy, like when a war ends and the casualties are tallied. Even though my former employer had no witnesses testify against me, it was difficult to separate this cold bureaucratic process from the hospital where I had worked. It was about numbers and money and politics and egos and turf. It wasn't about me, a human being, a valued ten-year employee. *How much is a body worth?*

A month later, I was on a Greyhound bus for a two-day, one-night trip from Denver to Sa-vannah for immunomodulatory treatment number ten. Even though I had won my work-ers' compensation suit six months before, I still hadn't seen one cent of my back pay. When I asked my lawyer, he said, "The judge has to sign the papers." How long could it take for a judge to sign his name to five pieces of paper? Six months and counting.

Raindrops on the roof of the bus beat out their staccato language. I paid admission to this darkened sideshow, was forced to look at what should not be seen. A stick-thin woman with a red dress and purple sweater and black fishnet stockings tried to pick up a black man, who was trying to mind his own business. The girl in the seat next to me asked, "Are we there yet?" I smiled and said, "No, soon."

In the chill morning, the driver smoked and talked to a shirtless man half hidden by the open door. Soon could mean before noon or within a year or two. Soon could mean never. Soon meant a hospital bed waited for me ahead. The narrow road swayed past as the world awakened to miles of cotton. The girl beside me once again slept. I envied an old woman sitting on her porch, her swing a cushion of stability. The future was rushing past too fast to grab hold. I slept on and off, feeling invisible. My watch lost time to the keening of tires.

Riding the bus through the south could best be described as "Hard Copy" meets "Hee-Haw." *The National Enquirer* on wheels. Scandals. Love triangles. Who was broke and who was kissing whom. The bus lurched over railroad tracks, past a broom and mop factory, along an orange-roped-off construction area. Behind me swirled Dolly Parton jokes, beauty tips, casserole recipes, and a litany of scandals about southern politicians. I marveled how southerners said two words when they could say one. They watered their flowers with hose pipe. Something happened each and every day. They named their sons Charlie Ray and their daughters Camellia Ann. A person suffered from yellow jaundice.

Nine-fifteen a.m. I was having a breakfast burrito and coffee in the bus depot. A black man came through the door from the street, looked around, and walked up to a black man sitting at a table. He placed a greenback in front of the man.

"Are you okay?" the man asked.

"I'm okay," the other man said.

"Great. I'm going to get a beer." The two men left the depot together and I made up a story in my mind about what I had just heard. "*The man was repaying his friend for a debt. The money on the table was a signal that a drug deal had just gone down. The man had just lost his wife and his friend has given him money for her funeral.*" Something in their lives made these men need beer before ten in the morning.

It was time to get back on the bus. The bus left without the men whose lives had touched mine in a desolate bus terminal. And once again I was grateful that, in these times that drive men away from inner contemplation, just as a forest fire drives a wild animal from his lair, I have the inner cave of writing where I can attempt to make sense of what I see, where I'm safe.

Are you okay? Yes, I'm okay.

⇌ ⇋

The bus pulled into Savannah, Georgia, at midnight. The only mode of transportation from Savannah to Hilton Head Island was by taxi. By the look of surprise on the driver's face, I knew he didn't get many fares to Hilton Head Island that originated from the bus station. On the thirty minute trip, he told me, in an accent so thick you could slather it like butter on bread, that he was recently divorced and a single father of a wayward fourteen-year-old daughter.

"I work twelve-hour shifts and just got out of the hospital last week because I got stabbed in the back. But that guy didn't have no luck," he said, with obvious satisfaction. "I put him in his coffin."

I really didn't care to investigate this line of conversation further, but it was obvious that my driver needed to talk, and so I listened. A guy had tried to rob him. In a low monotone, the driver explained that there had been a marked increase in crime, especially in the area around the bus station, especially at night. Wonderful. He certainly knew how to put a stranger at ease.

I arrived at the Emergency Room of Hilton Head Hospital about one a.m. They had a bed waiting. Actually, Room 220 was more like a suite, with its mauve-green-beige plaid cushions on a white wicker couch, glass-topped coffee table, two lamp tables with teal green lamps, and huge picture windows. Edna, the faithful night nurse, greeted me with a hug. After ten months of treatments, I was one of the regulars. We had shared life stories. She had held me when I cried.

Morning light brought towering pine trees and a blue South Carolina flag, with its white palmetto and white crescent moon insignias, waving outside my window. The usual rituals of consent form and subclavian insertion and fluoroscopy for catheter placement progressed smoothly. I knew the drill by heart. I was a veteran, a pro. The CVP catheter went smoothly into my left subclavian vein. Onward to the plasmapheresis room for the EKG monitor, the blood pressure checks, the usual routine.

Patti appeared with a Polaroid camera. "Dr. Medenica would like me to take a picture of you for a brochure he's having made about the plasmapheresis treatments. Is that okay with you?"

"Great. Now I'm a poster child for plasmapheresis," I groaned. "Do I get royalties?" Big laugh all around. They took 2,500 cc, 91 percent of my blood volume, out of my body and passed it through the machine, which separated plasma from white and red blood cells, filtered out the antigens, then sent it back into my body with new plasma. Plasmapheresis, that magenta circle, rolling into nowhere, so far from the end and so far from the beginning, like life—so hard to control. My prayer was that these treatments would bring a truce between my body and the foreign invader, allowing my body to cease fire and proclaim armistice, to enjoy lasting peace.

⁀ ⁀

"They're going to do a Utilization Review," my lawyer said during a long-distance phone call as I was finishing up treatment number ten. "They say that Dr. Medenica's treatment is experimental, but actually what they mean is that it's too expensive. They don't want to pay his bills." To the administrative judges, I was a certain percent of a whole person, price still to be determined, worth X percent of what I once was.

"The plasmapheresis has stopped the progress of the lupus. I was headed for a stroke before Dr. Medenica started treating me," I said. "Can they stop my treatments?"

"Yes, I'm afraid so," he replied.

The day of the Utilization Review, the judge ruled from the bench that Dr. Medenica would be allowed to continue as my treating physician. "Ms. Studer had received eight-plus years of 'traditional treatment' without benefit before she went to Medenica Clinic," he said. Lawyers for workers' compensation immediately appealed his decision.

June 1995. My case was argued before the Colorado Supreme Court. My lawyer was given fifteen minutes in which to present an oral argument stating the reasons Dr. Medenica should remain my treating physician. Six months later, the decision came down; the Colorado Compensation Authority would no longer pay for plasmapheresis treatments.

Twelve years after I became totally physically disabled, I filed a report with the Vaccine Adverse Reporting System about my Heptavax-B related illness. Finally, my story was one of the statistics gathering dust somewhere in the basement of the Food and Drug Administration. I was determined that, although my father's lobotomy so many years before had never been recorded, my story would be heard.

⇒ ⇐

My son was a six-foot-four man and scheduled to graduate from the University of Colorado the following week. He had earned a scholarship for his four years there from the Elks Club and had also worked very hard.

"Let's have lunch," Chris said over the phone. When he arrived, we caught up on his final exams and the latest girl he was dating. He pulled a small package out of his coat pocket.

"This is for you," he said, planting a kiss on my cheek. It was a tape of Bette Midler singing "Wind Beneath My Wings." "Did you ever know that you're my hero, everything I would like to be, you are the wind beneath my wings."

Chapter Ten
☞ TAMING THE WOLF ☜

I stopped my Datsun in front of the Rocky Mountain Pain Clinic on a sweltering summer day in 1984. I would rather have been doing anything else—taking a drive up Flagstaff Mountain or working on a poem or throwing a softball to my son—than be there. With a brick facade and glass display window, the clinic probably was a furniture store in a previous incarnation, but now, instead of displaying credenzas and rockers, there were stooped women and limping men on display. I opened the door and stepped into the waiting room. Even the potted fern seemed tense, its leaves straining toward the exit. The smell of disinfectant mingled with brewing coffee. Muzak dripped like water eroding rock—steady and unrelenting. Chrome was the dominant decor: tables, plant holders, picture frames. Vinyl cushions held nervous people as they leafed through *McCall's* or *Newsweek*.

The receptionist slid back the glass partition separating her from the patients, as if she was afraid that pain was contagious. "Would you please fill out the Pre-Treatment Psychological Test?" The glass door slammed shut.

I opened the booklet the same way I approached my yearly bout with the IRS. There were ten pages of thinly disguised inquiries into the health of my psyche:

1. You would rather be a social worker than a mountain climber. True or False.

2. You have recurrent fantasies of driving off a cliff or taking too many sleeping pills. True or False.

3. You are having a conflict with a coworker at your place of employment. Would you:

a. Ignore the person as much as possible.

b. Talk to your boss about the problem.

c. Set up an appointment with a third person to discuss the problem.

d. None of the above.

The gown was thin, the table hard, the room windowless, the air artificially chilled. After a year of dressing and undressing for strange doctors, I should have been used to the routine. But I wasn't. I shivered from my shoulders to my mottled toes. The exam table was raised, like a runway in a burlesque show. White paper crunched as I shifted weight to allow blood to flow to my feet. A neurologist, whom I had known when I worked in ICU, walked in. His expression told me how much I had changed, my slow gait, hesitant speech.

He slipped the Velcro blood pressure cuff around my arm. I was caught on the end of his tether. He asked me dates and times of the onset of symptoms and about hospitalizations at the University Hospital, at Presbyterian. He asked about blood tests, arteriograms, and biopsies. Again, I related the detours and highways of my medical odyssey: "Ill the day after I received the second dose of Heptavax-B vaccine…sore throat, aching muscles, rashes, hives that come and go…fast heart rate, blood in urine, high blood pressure…and by October…pain…dull in chest wall, in abdomen, with episodes of arterial spasm when fainting would be a relief…"

His pen crackled against the page. "Let me take a look," he said, washing his hands at the sink. He peered into my eyes with the ophthalmoscope, listened to my heart and lungs, palpated for the size of my liver and spleen, and drummed my knees, elbows, and ankles with a tiny steel hammer. Obediently, my body performed: legs bounced, chest heaved in and out like a bellows, pupils dilated and constricted on cue.

"You do have a problem," he said. "And by the way, I'm taking you off all your medications, including the pain medication, the prednisone, the cytoxin." The door snapped shut behind him before I could speak. In a letter to Dr. Shiovitz, Dr. S. wrote, "It's hard to believe that this woman is the same energetic nurse I used to see prancing around ICU."

⌒ ⌒

Seven-thirty to nine a.m. The pool. Like a schoolchild, I was herded onto the bus that carried the four women and five men in my group off to the warm, therapeutic pool. Undressing in the steamy locker room, I was forced to confront my body in the stark reality of four walls of mirrors. My cheeks were moon-round from months of taking prednisone. My hair had magically disappeared from under my arms and legs and pubic area. Hives dotted my cheeks and arms. My hands and feet were mottled. Easing into the warm pool, my body floated, weightless. I closed my eyes, floated on my back, once again graceful.

"Everyone in a circle now. Arms in front, now up, now down. Kick legs like a frog, one and two and three and four, all together in unison," our leader said.

Nine to nine forty-five a.m. Physical therapy. Retrieving a vinyl mat from the pile, I flopped down on top of it, along the perimeter of the ring, feet facing inwards, as if warming them at a fire.

"Hurts like hell," the woman next to me whispered. She wore a T-shirt that read "The Rooster Crows but the Hen Delivers."

"What did you say, Barbara? Remember, we don't want you talking about your pain with each other." The therapist stood in the center of the circle like a lion tamer wielding her whip. At her direction, we placed our hands on our abdomens, breathed deeply in, then out, stretched hip adductors and heel cords and hamstrings and low back and hip flexors. My feet went asleep from lack of circulation.

Ten to ten forty-five a.m. The psychologist. "Why can't I talk about my condition with the other people in this clinic? All the psychologists that I've heard of, from Kubler-Ross on down, say that talking about pain is one of the best ways of alleviating anger and stress," I asked.

"During the five years this clinic has been operating, we've found that, when people compare notes about injuries, it just reinforces pain behavior," he said.

"Pain behavior?" I asked. "What does that mean, pain behavior? I spend my days trying to rise above it, trying to get things done in spite of it, cooking meals, running the sweeper."

"That's good, tell me about it, tell me how you're doing," he said.

"Fine. Just fine." I looked at the books lining the walls behind his chair: *Anatomy of an Illness. Man and His Symbols. Mortal Lessons. Love, Medicine, and Miracles.*

Eleven to eleven forty-five a.m. Classes on stress reduction, nutrition, body mechanics. "Lie on your back, hands at your sides. Breathe in deeply, breathe out completely. You are in a forest, tall pines surround you on all sides. White light shines through the branches, shines down onto the top of your head, healing in its radiance…pain floats away on the beams of pure light…"

One to two-thirty p.m. Biofeedback. Tiny suction cups were placed on my forehead and arms and legs. The small Geiger counter-like machine on the table went crazy, beeping loudly, wire pointer bouncing within the red zone. Again, I was instructed to visualize a sandy beach or a magenta sunset.

"Those beeps remind me of the cardiac monitors in ICU where I used to work," I said. "A reminder that someone needs me, someone's life is in danger." When the technician turned down the sound, the pointer fell back into the safety zone, and I could relax. Each day, I took a nap while everyone else ate lunch.

The French philosopher René Descartes likened the human pain system to the bell-ringing apparatus of a church. The powerful tug of a burn or cut traveled along the rope of the neural pathway to the brain, where the alarm bell sounded and pain was perceived. When I worked in Intensive Care-Coronary Care as a registered nurse, I asked my patients to describe their pain on a scale of one to ten. Pain can be described in so many ways: fixed pain, migratory pain, deep pain, surface pain, stabs, throbs, burns. We human beings can walk on the moon but have not been able to defeat pain, our oldest enemy.

The four weeks I spent at the pain clinic gave me a new understanding of why the Latin word "poena" is also the word from which our English words "pain" and "punish" and "penalty" are derived. In this foreign world, pain was a behavior that was judged as to its validity, as to its worthiness for treatment. The clinic was a double bind experience. On the one hand, they told me to be independent and active in my care, but on the other hand, if I had a serious exacerbation, they wanted me to place myself submissively in their hands, and they would blame me for what I had done or failed to do that had worsened my symptoms.

One day a man erupted in anger and complained bitterly about being taken off his medications, before fleeing the building. By talking to the other patients, I learned that all of them were there because of work-related injuries, such as back pain or broken arms that hadn't healed properly. I was the only one there with a systemic illness that looked more and more like it was here to stay.

"Now just relax," Dr. Ben Tyler said, as he wiped my back with alcohol and pressed his fingers along my spine in search of the proper entry point. The spinal tap needle slid in effortlessly. He performed many tests that helped substantiate the toll the illness was taking on my body: "Neurological testing shows right hemisphere impairment; decreased motor skills, decreased reflexes." In his report, the psychologist wrote that I was handling my illness and all the uncertainties well, which was reassuring.

Within days of leaving the pain clinic, Dr. Shiovitz resumed my regimen of prednisone, cytoxin, and pain medicine. After many serious discussions about pain medications, he changed my pain medicine to Talwin.

"The vast majority of people who take narcotics for pain do *not* become addicts," he assured me. "Although tolerance (the requirement for bigger doses) and dependence (the development of withdrawal symptoms after sudden discontinuation) are associated with addiction, they do not represent true addiction by themselves."

Addiction is a condition in which people make obtaining and using the drug the centerpiece of their existence. The use of the drug becomes an end point in itself. Drug addicts withdraw from life and become less functional when they take drugs. In contrast, chronic pain patients become more functional when they use their drugs and are able to join in basic social activities frequently denied them by their pain. It is well established that chronic pain sufferers develop tolerance and dependence while on narcotics, but these are expected side effects—not signs of addiction—and are not considered indications for discontinuing the drug.

Tragically, tolerance and dependence are often mistaken for addiction, and the drugs are abruptly stopped. It is well known that pain patients sometimes take their own lives when their medications are discontinued. Some doctors call this phenomenon "algocide," suicide driven by pain. Patients with chronic pain are what make someone like Dr. Kevorkian possible.

⇌ ⇋

Chris, my heart walking outside my body, stood by the dining room table. He sucked his finger and then passed it quickly through the flame of the candle again and again. He was learning the trick of keeping his hand moving faster than fear, learning risk and consequence, mind over matter, faith over the luck of the draw. What made lightning single out one pulse in the middle of a crowd, turning light into a destructive force? The hand of God pointed at Job: "You are the one I have chosen for all this pain." How much should I tell Chris? I was the only parent he had. All my son knew was that his mother could unexpectedly end up in the hospital. He often found me lying in bed when he got home from school.

At fourteen, Chris was already five foot nine. He only owned two pairs of jeans, because every two months he was in a longer size. Suddenly, I was uncool. Oh, I could hang around like wallpaper but only so long as I wasn't too obvious. Eric and Kelly were cooler. Now his favorite music was nothing to which I could sing along. He called up his friends and arranged his social life and then later told me his plans. I was second-string, a bench-warmer for those nights when nobody else showed. He had one foot out my door. I loved hearing him hum, because one day soon he would be grown up and gone. The philosopher Aldous Huxley wrote about private universes or monads, within which each of us is eternally sealed. Even the brains of those whom we love the best—our mothers and lovers and sons—revolve in their solitary orbits around us.

＝ ＝

In Franz Kafka's novel *The Trial*, a passerby asked the hero, "How are you?" and he was paralyzed by being asked the one question he couldn't possibly answer. "How are you?" a friend would ask, and I had learned to offer a glib response. I knew he or she didn't want a report on the state of my kidneys or blood vessels or digestive dysfunction. Lupus means "wolf," and I kept trying to drive this wolf from my body. Some mornings I opened my bedroom door only to be surprised by the whole pack, a circle of snapping jaws, lightning lunges, driving me back into the dark safety of my house.

Then, out of nowhere came the unbridled laughter of my son, and his spirit made the wolf lie down, roll over, and play dead. The wolf turned into a pointy-nosed, tail-thumping, gently snoring pet that I got used to, like the sound of cicadas. Even though my veins spasmed and nerve endings twitched as I lay under the quilt, I learned to live with fear and what lay around its thin, ragged edges.

Against my will, I had been jettisoned to society's periphery—marginal, invisible. One of my mother's fundamentalist Christian friends said, "This is what God meant for you." A neighbor said, "God must really be impressed with you to throw such a big thing at you." Well-intentioned though these people were, these comments, meant to be encouraging, were difficult to hear. I maintained hope. I bargained for time while I fought with faith.

God and I circled in the ring under glaring lights. I tried jabs and tentative left hooks and right crosses that dissolved in midair. How to press an advantage, score a point, land a single punch? The audience on the periphery booed, then cheered. Bouts went on and on, round following round. Being a patient is a drama without words, an absolute experience, a public accounting of the innermost boundaries of a person's being. A patient enters the ring, intimate in near-nudity. A patient, like a boxer, brings every part of themselves to the fight. Everything is exposed, including secrets they don't even realize, the physical self, harmed cells, genetic codes. Medicine is the science of bruising with death, always a risk in this ring. A patient, like a boxer, must learn to exert will over the impulse to flee pain, to flee the unknown. A patient, like a boxer, is knocked out of time, leaving only the body's dialogue with its shadow self. The trick is turning wounds into wisdom. *"What is this pain telling me?"*

November 1992. My plasmapheresis and interferon treatments were done for another month, and I was discharged, dressed, and eating lunch when the pain in my belly began. I put on my call light. "What can we do for you?" a disembodied voice asked. Dr. Medenica had been successful in opening a clinic in Denver. He had gained approval to perform his immunomodulatory treatments at St. Anthony's Hospital. St. Anthony, the saint of dogs and cats.

"I'm having severe pain in my abdomen," I panted, "not like anything I've ever experienced before." Apart from the exquisite pain emanating from deep within, I was calm. Static serenity, as if the clock had stopped, my life frozen in this state of collapse. By the time a nurse arrived, I was moaning. "Can't you give me something?" I pleaded. The nurse checked my pulse, cool fingers against my carotid, her eyes fixed on her wristwatch.

"Dr. Medenica has already left for South Carolina," the nurse said. "I'll have to make some calls." She left. I shut my eyes and saw my son's shining face. Nausea rushed up like a wave from abdomen to face, sweat pearled my temples. As long as I lay perfectly still and quietly allowed the nurses to take my blood pressure, the pain was bearable.

I pretended I was floating on the ocean, breathing with care. *Concentrate. Be calm.* The face of the ER doctor appeared. I felt his hand on my abdomen. He left. The nurses inserted a Levin tube, a plastic tube snaking from nose to stomach. Another strange doctor appeared, and this time he read my chart. A gurney was brought in and set parallel to my bed as a circle of faces formed above me.

"I'm not a complainer," I gasped to one of the nurses.

"We know that, Connie," she said, holding my hand. Hospitals usually err on the side of caution. Delay in treating her patient's agony might never get a nurse in trouble, but her death surely would.

An LPN appeared and held my hand. Another doctor came and felt my abdomen, which was guarded, getting hard. Agony didn't begin to describe how I felt. My dear friend Morgan walked into my room like a guardian angel. I hadn't known she was coming. She had decided at the last moment. *"Thanks,"* I said to her with my eyes. In a silent language that true friends share, she understood how badly I needed help.

How do you measure pain? As a nurse, I remember patients who were labeled drug addicts because they had the bell on for their shot before it was time. I had learned as a nurse to ask patients, "How bad is your pain on a scale of one to ten?" and judged a person a three because their fists weren't clenched. Now I knew that pain could be off any scale man could invent. Seven hours later, I was wheeled into the operating room.

Light swam on the ceiling. The sound of voices faded in and out. Farther away, a woman yelled, another laughed. A lot of instruments hummed, clicked, flashed, thumped. I was propped on my side with pillows behind my back and between my legs. I felt no pain. *"Is my body there? Why is it so noisy?"* I wondered. Then I remembered.

The perforation, the emergency surgery. The surgeon stood by my bed. I concentrated on his stethoscope looped around his wrist, while his large thumbs were hooked under the waistband of his scrubs. My eyes swam into focus as I lifted my head. Blue drapes framed soft cracks of light. I slept. Later, I saw my friend Ruth's face close to mine. Then Chris was standing next to my bed.

"Hi, sweetheart," I said.

He walked closer to my bed. "Hey, Mom. How you doing?"

"Did I have the operation?" I asked.

"You did," he replied.

"I feel like I'm floating in space." A nurse approached with a thermometer. I heard a respirator and knew I was in ICU. As if on cue, Chris waved and backed out of the room. I felt the electrodes on my chest as the cardiac monitor blinked on my right. Dried spittle pasted the corners of my mouth together. I was a mess.

Later that day, I was transferred to a surgical floor. *Dangle feet. Sit on side of bed.* I had to walk today. Easy. A cinch. Brown hair wild, uncombed. Knobby knees, weak feet wobbling in scruffy slippers. Striped hospital gown open in the back, everything exposed. Who cared? A nurse provided a bathrobe. IV pole tottering along behind, I started down the hall to the solarium. Fragile. Stitches pulled. *Stand straight. Deep breath.*

I had a ten-inch midline, new, raw opening that extended from sternum to below the navel. That is what "exploratory surgery" means; "We open you up wide and look around and repair what's broken." I knew the numbness of those who have seen too much, the soldier returning permanently scarred. Scar tissue, that map to the past. Emotionally, too, I was on the bottom and was surprised to find it solid. I spent the next ten days in St. Anthony's Hospital recuperating from emergency surgery, just another saga in the medical history of Connie Studer, retired nurse, itinerant writer.

Once home, I avoided visits from anyone but calm, close kin and proven friends who asked few questions, gave no predictions, and made no demands. More stunned than despairing, I was unable to write a word. I lay in my bed watching leaves sway on trees and looked no further ahead than what I would cook for dinner.

I always thought I was a compassionate nurse, but until I lay in the hospital bed myself, was given the wrong medication, and was treated badly by an arrogant doctor, I had no idea what patients went through. Care of the sick, like meditation or prayer, demands immersion in the moment. In life, just as in writing a poem, I had to learn how to layer pain in metaphors and emotions so that I could take it in. Layer it like the stroke of fingers on an arm, like the stanzas in a psalm. Intuition, like poems, came from electricity in the air, a hum inside, impulses felt deep within the body.

Illness was my wake-up call to identify what was truly important. The power of thinking positively, support groups, lifestyle changes. Disability was a balancing act, where every step meant leaving one safe foothold to reach for another. When the leader of my support group asked us to talk about the benefits of our illnesses, I was startled. However, answers came from around the room: "I appreciate my loved ones more;" "I argue less;" "I appreciate every moment of the day much more." Using guided imagery, she assisted me, along with the others, in shifting our focus from fear of sickness and death to motivation for self-improvement. Physical problems were a given. True health was how I learned to deal with them.

Living with lupus was like inheriting a large mirror where I had gotten used to the face looking back every morning, but a thief entered my house while I was away on vacation. I returned to find the mirror smashed in thousands of pieces against the hearth. The rest of my life would be spent trying to glue slivers onto a black canvas. I prayed that someday the mirror would once again shimmer with color and strength.

Pain is one chord sung from deep in the heart, sprung from the back of the throat and belly, where all songs are born. Like John the Baptist screaming from the woods or Job bemoaning his boils or Blake in his eternal moment, the blood-pulse making heaven out of moon, sun, man. *Leave me alone. Don't leave me alone. Let me be this stone skipped on moontide. Let me be light on water. Let me save myself.*

Chapter Eleven

⮎ Twice Born ⮌

My mother saw gremlins. The house was crowded with babies only she could feed and boyfriends vying for the pleasure of taking her out for a milkshake. Parkinson's disease had taken hold eight years before, and now she struggled to stay attached at brain-root and tongue-stem.

"Just have enough faith, and you'll be healed," my mother had told me back in 1984, when I went on disability from the hospital where I had worked for ten years. But, in spite of her fervent prayers, Mother began having increased difficulty walking. My sister Kathy had taken over our mother's care, a heavy load. Eventually, both my mother and sister were faced with the reality of an unrelenting, downward progression after a succession of Parkinson's medications no longer helped.

"Here's the doctor's number and our neighbor's number if you need help," Kathy said. "This is where I'll be." Already she had her suitcase in hand, one foot out the door. I was back in my mother's home in Georgia, in the summer of 1991. I had volunteered to take care of our mother for a week so that my sister, who had been a toddler when I left home to enter nurse's training, could have a much-needed vacation.

"I'm late," Mother said, her pupils large with anxiety. "Charlie's here a lot, always wanting money, but now he smiles at me. Once he even said he was sorry. Do you know where Daddy took the babies?"

Her legs contracted in spasms, bouncing her almost out of her wheelchair. Another moment and I would have to pick her up. I stood, locked knees with her, and scooted her back onto the chair.

"What babies?" I asked.

"The little girls," she replied. Maybe in her mind she saw Pat and me helping her weed our garden or Barbara or Kathy or Jeanne when they were still toddlers. Or maybe it was Marguerite, my sister, who had died at eight months from spina bifida. Or maybe she was back on the farm where she was raised and watching over her little sister, Kathryn. Or maybe she was worried about herself surviving on the Ohio dirt farm where she was born.

"It doesn't help to contradict her reality," my sister had told me. "He'll have them back in time for bed," I assured her. Carefully, I read the instructions that my sister had left, the times and dosages of eight medicines she gave my mother every day, Mother's daily regime, her food preferences;. "Up on commode. Brush teeth. Help her downstairs ten steps to kitchen, one-half grapefruit. Corn flakes. Pills. Commode. Sponge bath. Clean sweats and shirt. Help her with the walker back to her reclining chair. Commode. Pills. Commode. Down on the couch for a nap. Pills. Commode. In front of TV for dinner."

This was the same woman who had cooked countless Thanksgiving feasts. The woman who had learned how to water ski on Lake Hartwell when she was well into her sixties, even though she sped around the lake stooped over, always in danger of falling. The woman who had taught Bible verses to neighborhood children. As a nursing supervisor, I had kept a whole hospital running through a ten-hour shift. Surely that was more difficult than caring for one elderly woman.

When I awakened at three a.m. to give her the Sinemet, Mother was lying on the floor next to her bed.

"I'm just across the hall," I said. "Why didn't you call me?"

"Didn't want to bother you," she said impishly. "That man will help us."

"There's no man here," I replied. "Just us chickens. Okay, let's get you back into bed." Knees braced, slowly I pulled her up, both of us struggling to retain balance. The rigidity caused by her disease was compounded by the fact that she was actively resisting my attempts to help her stand. Hurriedly, I cantilevered her down onto the commode before I lost my balance, too. She laughed as she landed with a plop. Like a child, her face lit up as she peed, looking at me for approval. Now I was the parent, and she was my child.

"Do you see Daddy lying there on the bed?" my mother asked with a coquettish smile. Dad Browne had been dead for twenty years, Dad Adams for twenty-seven. It wasn't clear to whom she was referring.

"No, Mama, I don't," I said.

"We're getting along better than we ever have," she replied.

"Why is that?" I asked.

"Because he doesn't talk back to me anymore," she said. "How does my sister do this, day in, day out?" I wondered. There has to be a special place in heaven reserved for caretakers of the elderly.

⌐ ⌐

In *The Varieties of Religious Experience*, the philosopher William James spoke of two kinds of practical personal perspectives on experience, which he characterized as the once and twice born. The once born were described as naive optimists who tended to see everyday life and religion on the surface: hopeful, positive, well-ordered, progressive. The twice born, in contrast, were more pessimistic and tended to focus on the darker underside of experience. The twice born were absorbed by questions of social injustice and personal pain. The experience of chronic illness often converts the once born into the twice born.

Why me? Why am I sick? Because you've been bad. But how do I know I've been bad? Because you're sick. The less medical science knew about an illness—lupus, for instance—the more sickness was considered a character flaw, a sickness of the soul or a personality defect or a moral deformity. In my experience, doctors and nurses are decent men and women doing their best against impossible odds.

When I moved to Boulder in 1973, it was a bustling hub for pathways to not only good health, but also salvation. Fundamentalist Christians were convinced that illness was a punishment from God for sin. The worse the illness, the more unspeakable the sin must have been. Adherents to New Age dogma said, "You are giving yourself this disease because there is something important you must learn for your spiritual growth." They believed that the mind alone caused illness and that the mind alone could cure it. Western doctors said illness was a biophysical disorder caused by viruses or trauma or genetic predispositions. Eastern doctors said illness represented the burning up and purifying of a past misdeed. Psychologists said repressed emotions caused illness—illness as death wish. Or maybe illness was only an illusion, like the Gnostics said, "Spirit is the only reality, and in spirit there is no illness." Holistic doctors said illness was the product of physical, emotional, mental, and spiritual factors all together. Buddhists said illness was inescapable, like air. Only through enlightenment could illness be transcended.

Early one morning in January 2000, I received a call from Kathi Williams at the National Vaccine Information Center. "Would you be willing to give a statement in front of the Committee on Health and Welfare at the Colorado House of Representatives? There is a bill that Representative Shawn Mitchell has proposed to remove hepatitis B from the list of mandatory immunizations in the state of Colorado."

"Yes, I'd be happy to," I said. "When?"

"Next Monday," she replied.

"I'll be there."

The chamber at the Colorado courthouse had salmon-colored walls and stained glass windows depicting early settlers, Native Americans, trains, and majestic mountains. Representative Mitchell rose to present his arguments for this bill. "Hepatitis B is different from other immunizations because hepatitis B is an adult disease," he said. "It isn't right to expose every infant and child in our state to the possibility of adverse effects. Between 1990 and 1995, there were only six children in Colorado who came down with hepatitis B infections. Why expose all of our children to the risks of serious illnesses that can be caused by this vaccine?"

Those in opposition to Representative Mitchell's bill spoke first. The Chief Medical Officer of the Department of Public Health said he opposed the bill because "vaccinations help young children prepare for life. We are as concerned as anyone about safety. Rotavirus is an example of a vaccine that when problems were recognized was quickly taken off the market. There is no scientifically researched evidence at this point that there are any serious adverse effects to the hepatitis B vaccine."

In July 1999, The Advisory Committee on Immunization Practices (ACIP) had suspended RotaShield (Wyeth Laboratories) after fifteen cases of intussusception, a telescoping of the intestines causing bowel obstruction, were reported to the Vaccine Adverse Event

Reporting System (VAERS). The vaccine had been developed as a protection for infants and young children against severe diarrhea.

"Does your office record adverse reactions, sir?" the chairwoman asked.

"Adverse reactions are filed with the CDC and the FDA," he replied "We don't get a report specific to Colorado cases back."

"Then you don't really know how many adverse events to the hepatitis B vaccine there have been in Colorado, do you?" she asked.

"No, I agree that we need a Colorado database of adverse effects." He finished and sat down. Ten other people stood to testify in favor of the mandatory immunization of children in our state, even though thimerosal, a form of mercury used as a preservative, had recently been banned from use in vaccine production. However, the removal of thimerosal was not mandatory, merely a recommendation to the pharmaceutical companies. Yes, it was true that doctors didn't have any incentive to report adverse events and that any reporting to the pharmaceutical company or to the FDA was not mandatory but voluntary. Yes, they admitted that there was a strong profit motivation, from both the federal and state governments, to support the immunization programs in place.

Next, those of us opposed to giving hepatitis B vaccine to all Colorado children had our chance to speak. Drs. Incao and Orient made the point that, "First of all, doctors must do no harm." Patients should be treated as individuals, instead of as part of a herd. The lack of informed consent protections in mass vaccination programs are leading to fear and mistrust of the whole vaccination system. "Parents are saying, 'Show us the science and give us a choice,'" Dr. Incao said.

"There were 24,775 hepatitis B vaccine-related events reported to the Vaccine Adverse Reporting System (VAERS) in all age groups, including 9,673 serious adverse events and 439 deaths between July 1, 1990 and October 31, 1998. Out of this total, 17,497 reports were in individuals who received only hepatitis B vaccine," he continued.

In 1993, a former FDA Commissioner wrote in the *Journal of the American Medical Association* that one study showed "only about 1 percent of serious events attributable to drug reactions are reported to the FDA."

Professor Bonnie Dunbar, Ph.D., a Texas cell biologist and a vaccine-research pioneer, rose to speak. "It takes weeks and sometimes months, for autoimmune disorders, such as rheumatoid arthritis, to develop following vaccination. No basic science research or controlled, long-term studies into the side effects of this vaccine have been conducted in American babies, children, or adults. We need informed consent for hepatitis B vaccinations, as well as National Institute of Health funding for independent research, to determine the biologic mechanism for hepatitis B vaccine reactions in order to identify high-risk factors and to develop therapies to repair vaccine damage."

Barbara Loe Fisher, co-founder of the National Vaccine Information Center, gave testimony: "Newborn babies are dying shortly after their shots and their deaths are being written off as sudden infant death syndrome. Parents should have the right to give their informed consent to vaccination and Congress should give emergency, priority funding to independent scientists, who can take an unbiased look at this vaccine, instead of leaving the research in the hands of government officials, who have already decided to force every child to get the vaccine."

Finally, it was my turn. I stood at the podium, legs quaking but voice strong and told my story. "Madame Chairman, Members of the Committee, thank you for this opportunity to speak to you in support of this bill. I am a retired registered nurse and a writer. I received Heptavax-B, an attenuated virus vaccine made by Merck, Sharp, and Dohme in 1983, while working as a nursing supervisor at a local hospital. My serious reaction has been a life-altering, catastrophic illness. I had been a registered nurse for twenty years, had worked in an Intensive Care-Coronary Care unit, then as evening supervisor of the hospital. After the second dose of this vaccine, I became increasingly ill, then totally disabled in 1984. After many biopsies, consultations with specialists, hospitalizations, and treatments, I was diagnosed as having systemic lupus erythematosus, systemic vasculitis, and glomerulonephritis, induced by the hepatitis B vaccine. I have gone from being an active woman to one who spends her days living with chronic pain, who must pace activities in order to continue living independently.

"Hepatitis B is an adult disease which is not highly contagious, is not deadly for most who contract it, and is not in epidemic form in the United States. Little is known about the health and integrity of an individual baby's immune and neurological systems at birth. If my middle-aged immune system could not tolerate the vaccine, how can a few-days-old baby's immune system?

"In 1986, the United States Congress passed the National Childhood Vaccine Injury Compensation program because parents were suing pharmaceutical companies because of injuries to their children. This compensation program was instituted in order to protect pharmaceutical companies from lawsuits. In 1994, a book entitled *Adverse Events Associated With Childhood Vaccines* was published by the Institute of Medicine. The fourteen physician-authors spend 347 pages to say, 'We don't know if vaccines cause chronic illness because no one has ever studied it.' No one has followed up on patients, like me, who suffered serious adverse effects. Who would fund such research? The pharmaceutical companies would never fund a study that might incriminate their own product, laying them open for litigation. Why doesn't the FDA fund this research, since they are the ones responsible for the Vaccine Adverse Event Reporting System (VAERS)? Why isn't it mandatory for doctors to inform patients of the risks of immunizations, just as they must before performing an appendectomy or a spinal tap?

"It was twelve years after becoming totally physically disabled that I filed a VAERS report about my vaccine-related illness. Finally, I was one of the statistics gathering dust somewhere in the basement of the FDA. Is it any wonder that it's so difficult to make a clear connection between vaccines and chronic illnesses, such as lupus? If it happens to you or your child, the risk is 100 percent. Thank you."

The last person to speak was a woman who lived in Vail with her husband and three-year-old son. She testified that her son had been a normal baby when she took him for his seven-month, well-baby checkup. The pediatrician gave the baby a hepatitis B vaccine, the only vaccine he received that day. Within four hours, the baby had a high fever and was crying inconsolably. The frantic mother had called for an ambulance, but by the time the ambulance got there, the baby was in a coma. He was on life support in a pediatric intensive care for months. Slowly, he awoke, but this woman's three-year-old son now had the intellectual development of a one-year-old child. The doctors told Kirsten and her husband that their son was permanently brain-damaged, but none of the doctors were willing to say that this damage was caused by the hepatitis B vaccine. Therefore, this family could not file a claim with the National Federal Vaccine Injury Compensation program. "We need to ask more questions, demand more answers," she said.

The bill that would have eliminated the hepatitis B vaccine from all mandatory vaccines prescribed for every Colorado child did not pass this committee. It was determined that there would be further discussion with "health care professionals in a health care task force." The Chairman felt "uncomfortable in changing policy." Of course, to "postpone indefinitely" was politician-speak for killing the bill.

Six hours after the hearing began, we filed out of the chamber and gathered in clusters, consoling each other. Kirsten stood crying in her husband's arms. Her son stared into space and drummed his foot on the floor. She bent down and scooped her son up into her arms.

⌒ ⌒

"Come now," Kathy's voice said on my answering machine. "Mama's gone. I love you." I sat on the floor and placed both palms over my heart, as if I were holding a bandage trying to stop bleeding. I thought I was prepared for this. My mother had said good-bye to me six years earlier when she could still speak. Now it was 1997, and my mother was gone, and I had to be with her. My brain had every wire crossed.

"Grandma died," I said to Chris over the phone. Through the back door, the leaves on the ash shimmered in a long rush of wind.

"I'll come with you. Are you okay?" he asked.

"I haven't cried yet. Isn't that strange?" I replied.

"Do you want me to come over?" he said.

"No. I'll make the arrangements. See you tomorrow at the airport, honey. Thanks." I booked two tickets and threw clothes into the suitcase without thinking about matching colors or preventing wrinkles. A song played over and over in my brain: "And a rock feels no pain; And an island never cries."

Georgia humidity clung to my skin like cellophane. The countryside was an Eden of kudzu, pines, and hickories. Pat was at the house already. Kathy greeted us, looking exhausted. Barbara and Charlie flew in from Ohio. Jeanne and her family drove from West Virginia.

Walking through my mother's house, I saw that nothing had changed. There was the same green blanket thrown over the gold couch, the coffee table with its orange and red plastic flowers, the piano laden with graduation portraits. Dad Browne's marble-topped Victorian tables held stained glass lamps. A picture of Jesus smiled benevolently from the wall.

I stood at the kitchen window of my mother's home, my hands lost in soapy dishwater, my mind far away: *I'm sitting on the broad backs of workhorses. Cornstalks wave like fans. I'm eating a bowl of popcorn after school, because Mama won't be home until late.* Through the door, I heard Barbara and Charlie on the patio talking and smoking. Laughter washed in through the screen door, along with the odor of rusty metal and sweet wet grass. I opened the refrigerator, retrieved a soda, and joined my family outside. Chris waved me to a seat next to him.

"What kinds of flowers should we order?" Jeanne asked.

"Mom liked lilies," Pat said, "and roses."

"I brought pictures of Mom and Dad Browne and Dad Adams to display at the funeral home," I said.

"Good," Kathy said. "We won't have to worry about food. Women from church brought enough casseroles and salads to last a week. They're going to provide a dinner at the church after the funeral."

"I'll never forget all those huge dinners Mom prepared—ham and turkey and four vegetables and five desserts," Pat said. She loved to see people fall away from her table, begging for mercy."

"She made most of our clothes growing up," I said. "She used to kneel at my feet, her mouth full of pins, unpicking her tiny stitches, doing them over until they were perfect."

"Did you know that Mom was engaged to someone named Norman Swinehart before she married Lucien, but she broke it off?" Jeanne asked. "'I just couldn't marry the common man,' she said."

Pat and Kathy retreated to the kitchen; soon there was the clatter of dishes being washed and dried. Once again I merged into the family fold, the hubbub of people to whom I was connected by blood and circumstance. Charlie sat smoking in the recliner that had been our mother's throne. I walked through her house, running my hands over the familiar desk and piano and needlepoint rug that Dad Browne had created.

Barbara picked through a box of photos. Ghosts of our relatives sifted through her hands. She handed me a picture of two toddlers standing on either side of a basket of flowers, Pat and I in white nurses' outfits that our mother had made, complete with white caps and red crosses on our sleeves. Our father's smile beamed through the bouquet. Under the photos, there was a yellow newspaper clipping that read, "Infant Daughter Dies in Adams Home. Marguerite Joanne Adams, infant daughter of the Reverend and Mrs. Lucien Adams, passed away at her home in Whitehouse on Saturday evening, August 17. She was born January 9, 1946 at Lodi Hospital. Besides her parents, she is survived by two sisters, Patricia Ann and Constance Elaine." No pictures exist of Marguerite. My family was too poor to own a camera.

"Is this you, Connie?" Kathy asked, holding up a photo of a little girl sitting cross-legged under a large tree. She wore a cowboy hat, a flannel shirt, and jeans, with a look of defiance in her eyes.

"Afraid so," I said, inspecting the picture more closely. "I must have been about six. This is the backyard of the farmhouse in Elmore that Mama rented after our father went into Toledo State Hospital. I loved that old farmhouse. It had a large front porch and that wonderful barn where I used to swing on a rope from one haymow to the other."

"Did Mom know you did that?" Kathy asked.

"Don't think so," I said. "It's just as well."

Jeanne, the musician in the family, sat down at the piano and leafed through the hymnal. Under her fingers, the piano became a mournful voice: "I come to the garden alone, while the dew is still on the roses…"

The undertaker arrived to discuss the funeral arrangements with Kathy: choosing a casket, hours for visitation at the funeral home, the bulletin for the service, burial at the cemetery afterwards. The sky rumbled and rain fell softly, cooling everything down. Rain on the grass and lilacs and pinecones released a sweet smell. Georgia rain was softer than Colorado rain, like the difference between velvet or denim brushing my skin.

As we sat around the table heavy with ham and date nut bread and Waldorf salad, I looked at my middle-aged siblings. Charlie still had his red hair but was short and stocky and wheezed from emphysema. Barbara was golden with her short blond hair, gorgeous smile, and gold and diamond jewelry. Pat's many years as a Methodist minister's wife gave her a calm, dignified air but also a great sense of humor. Kathy had the elfin look of Leslie Caron. Jeanne, the youngest, was thin, with the long blond hair of a Jean Seberg. *"Why has it taken us twenty years to be together in our mother's home?" I wondered.*

Later, at the funeral home, Mother, always the most alive of women, lay in a gray casket in her sea-green suit, small as a child against the ivory cushion. Her hair was still dark brown, with streaks of silver. She died three weeks shy of her eightieth birthday. Her left hand was curled up tight with contractures that refused to relax, even in death.

The day we buried Mother, the air was filled with honeysuckle, sweet alyssum, and magnolias, all those southern flowers brewed into a humid soup. One by one, my brother, sisters, nieces, nephews, and my son emerged from the bedrooms ready to depart for the church. The low brick Christian and Missionary Alliance Church stood with its doors flung open as people filed into the dim interior. Mother's children followed solemnly behind her casket. The minister stood behind the pulpit and raised his arms. "'I am the resurrection and the life,' saith the Lord; 'he that believeth in me, though he were dead, yet shall he live: and whosoever liveth and believeth in me shall never die.'" His voice was hopeful and strong. Mike, a Baptist minister and Jeanne's husband, gave a eulogy for the family, praising my mother's energy, her skill in the kitchen, and her missionary zeal. We rose for the recessional and followed our mother back down the aisle. I shut my eyes against the sun, and finally, tears came.

The last time I saw Mother alive was the summer before she died. By that time, my mother lived in her bedroom. As hard as Kathy tried, the odor of urine rose from the room like smoke. Mother lay on her bed, draped in a blue cotton nightgown, reduced to a breathing skeleton. She could not speak. No one knew how much she understood, if anything. Curled in the fetal position, her eyes were open but unseeing, her skin bruised and sallow, her hands contracted into claws. There was no sign she was alive until Kathy touched her. At the lightest touch, Mother shrieked, whether in pain or fear it, was impossible to know. She hadn't talked in three years or walked in four. She was a prisoner in her own body, in a twilight zone, vegetative state. There were no comforting answers to this tragedy before me on the bed. Withdrawing nutrition would be active euthanasia, but who would want to live like this?

I lifted my mother to change her diaper. Sun broke through the window, reflecting tree branches against the wall. Mother's bones were sharp against my chest, her body thinned to this shaking weight. Her eyes were closed. I wanted her suffering to be over. I wanted to hold her in this world even though she had already said "Good-bye, I love you." Her hair, still brown and soft, brushed my cheek. I laid her back on the sheet. My shoulders were work-sore, and I felt that first weight in my chest that I would later recognize as grief. All that was left of Mother was moist breath against the pillowcase and small sighs and a fading physical form. I could still hear her saying "Stand up straight, study hard. If you put the 'umph' in 'try,' you get 'triumph.'" I leaned back on air as if my mother were still holding me up.

Chapter Twelve
☞ BODY LANGUAGE ☜

"Cry now, or every loss is your mother all over again," one of Mother's Georgia friends said to me at her funeral. Even months later, back home in Colorado, I awoke each morning with *"It's true"* roaring through my head. All attempts at sympathy brought on sulks. I cried for my mother when I banged my knee or had a disagreement with a friend or couldn't make up my mind what to do next. I carried on imaginary conversations with her:

"I wish you were here, Mama."

"You know I'm better off now. Now you don't have me trying to run your life."

"I'm jealous of anyone who still has her mother."

"I know, dear."

It is difficult to approach the memory of my mother head-on. Always she has been too central, a powerful force in my life. She returns to me in fragments, when I hear church bells or smell pink roses or beat eggs with a fork. I feel her in my hands. "God exalts no one but the humble," she used to say. Humble my mother was not, but I had seen how, even though life brought her down, she never gave up. Mother taught me that a woman must know how to take care of herself and that having enough money for food and shelter was the most sincere form of love. The greatest legacy I received from my resourceful mother was learning to face my problems, whether I wanted to or not. She taught me to become an active participant in life rather than merely a survivor, how to make choices and to live with the consequences. As I fall asleep at night after a particularly exhausting day, I dangle my hand over the side of the bed and feel another hand touch mine. The warmth remains.

After I moved to Boulder, my sister, Pat, visited Chris and me often. Over and over, we dissected our family history as sun streamed through the front window of my little home, Pat on one couch and me on the other, cups of coffee warming our hands. She was the person who had also experienced the many facets of our mother's complex personality: the charming social butterfly, the evangelistic preacher, the grief-stricken wife visiting her husband in a mental hospital, the strict disciplinarian. Pat was the sister who understood when I separated from my husband and kept me company on the three-day journey west. Many years later, she told me that her return home to Ohio was the first time she had ever flown in an airplane. Together, my sister and I often affirmed and sometimes disputed each other's perceptions of reality. But it was by talking about our past that both of us learned to accept our family history. *Could our mother have done more? Why did she sign the consent form for our father's lobotomy?*

"Remember when Mr. Rader brought a puppy for you on Christmas Eve and how upset Mama was, but she couldn't say no because it was a Christmas gift?" Pat asked.

"I named him Buddy," I said. "How I loved him. And then one day he just disappeared."

"You never knew what happened to him?" she asked.

"No.," I replied. "Mama said she gave him away because he was killing the neighbor's chickens."

"He got hit by the school bus," Pat said.

"What? How do you know?" I asked.

"Mama and I found him in the middle of the road. Mama told me not to tell you," Pat replied. "It wasn't very long after Daddy went into the hospital. Do you ever wonder what our father's life was like after his surgery?"

"I've got a good idea. I went to see him while I was in nurse's training," I said.

"You did? When?" she asked.

"Toledo State Hospital was part of our psychiatric rotation. I read his chart and copied down a lot of it. He didn't know me and ran toward me, as if he wanted to hurt me. It was awful. For a long time I didn't want to admit that my father was in a mental hospital. I'm sorry I didn't go with you to his funeral. I let you down."

"All is forgiven," my sister said, with a hug.

⌒ ⌒

The human brain is the ultimate *terra incognita,* the last frontier. Lobotomy, the only medical procedure formally condemned by the Vatican and banned in Russia, was what turned my father's life into monitored trips to the bathroom, games of checkers, and clothing forever lost. The tragedy of lobotomy was its irreversibility once the deed was done.

The gothic tale of lobotomy was one of hubris and megalomania and greed. Center stage in this tragic play were Dr. Ugo Cerletti, an Italian professor of psychiatry, Dr. Egaz Moniz, a Portuguese neurologist, and Dr. Walter Freeman, an American neuropathologist and neuropsychiatrist.

While visiting a slaughterhouse, Dr. Cerletti observed how hogs became more docile after electric current surged through their temples; he saw the possibility for applying this therapy to his patients. All that energy ignited his entrepreneurial spirit—so many medical and financial possibilities. In 1935, Dr. Egaz Moniz performed the first prefrontal lobotomy, for which he was awarded the Nobel Prize for Physiology/Medicine in 1949, a prize he shared with Walter Hess. In 1939, Dr. Moniz was shot and paralyzed by one of his lobotomized patients who was unhappy with his surgery. In 1955, at the age of eighty-one, he was beaten to death in his office by another dissatisfied lobotomized patient.

It was Dr. Walter Freeman who, after observing Dr. Moniz's surgery in Spain, brought lobotomy to the United States in 1936. With evangelistic zeal, Freeman stated that he intended to empty out the back wards of mental hospitals. Although he had no training in surgery, Dr. Freeman traveled from mental hospital to mental hospital, performing lobotomies without gloves or anesthesia. An ordinary ice pick became his most economical and expedient surgical tool. He recommended transorbital lobotomy for diagnoses ranging from psychosis to depression to neurosis to criminality.

By 1945, ten children between the ages of four and six had undergone lobotomy "to smash the world of fantasy in which they were enslaved," Dr. Freeman said. One of the arguments that Freeman used to gain entrance to back ward patients was the high incidence of suicide among electroshock and insulin-shock patients. Since this high mortality rate cast psychiatrists in a bad light, Freeman promised to lower this suicide rate because lobotomy created "wax dummies," "china-doll phenomenon." *Sit them up and their eyes open; lay them down and their eyes close.*

When eventually some doctors questioned Freeman's techniques and results, he reluctantly accepted Dr. Watts, a surgeon, as his partner. Together, Drs. Freeman and Watts, cochairmen of the Department of Neurology and Neurological Surgery at George Washington University, self-published *Psychosurgery: Intelligence, Emotion and Social Behavior* (1942). The dust jacket bore the following blurb: "Read the last chapter to find out how those treasured frontal lobes, supposed to be man's most precious possession, can bring him to psychosis and suicide! …Here for the first time certain intellectual processes are revealed as running along with emotion, when the connection between the frontal lobe and the thalamus is severed… This work reveals how personality can be cut to measure, sounding a note of hope for those who are afflicted with insanity."

This book contains transcripts of the conversations between Freeman and his patients during the operation. Because the patients only received a local anesthetic, it was possible to document progressive changes in the patient's mental state as the operation proceeded.

The book stated: "Unresponsiveness or disorientation are usually necessary in order to obtain a satisfactory clinical result. When euphoria, not associated with other intellectual change [unresponsiveness and disorientation] is present within a few days after lobotomy, a relapse usually occurs."[1]

Dr. Freeman called his forays across America promoting lobotomy "head-hunting expeditions" and referred to his patients as "trophies." His standard fee for the ten-minute surgery was one thousand dollars. He didn't believe in all that "germ crap" and once performed a lobotomy on a motel room floor. When even his partner, Dr. Watts, finally balked at performing the transorbital or ice pick lobotomies, Dr. Freeman instructed those lower on the totem pole of medicine, aides or orderlies, on the fine art of brain surgery.

There is an old saying in medicine that you should neither be the first nor the last to start using a new drug or procedure. However, being part of the medical crowd's collective judgment is often based more on enthusiasm than on scientific evidence. In fact, after a certain critical mass of doctors have adopted a practice, such as lobotomy or immunizations, the physicians can be more legally vulnerable by shunning the procedure, since the "standard of practice" they'll be measured against in a court of law is precisely what their colleagues are currently doing.

The popular press jumped on the lobotomy bandwagon. "Surgery Used on the Soul-Sick; Relief of Obsessions is Reported," was a *New York Times* headline. "Pluck from the brain a hidden sorrow," a 1940 article in *The Medical Record* said. *Time* reported, "The surgeon's knife can reach into the brain and sever the tensions which underlie a psychopathic personality." "Patients are encouraged to sing and pray... No worse than a tonsillectomy," the newspapers stated. Even prominent, wealthy families like the Kennedys did not escape lobotomy. When Rosemary Kennedy, who was mildly mentally retarded, expressed interest in boys, her father, Joseph Kennedy, had her institutionalized and gave consent for a lobotomy to be performed on his daughter. Even though she was never mentally ill, the famous but eccentric actress Frances Farmer was admitted to a psychiatric hospital and received a lobotomy.

In the fall of 1941, the American Medical Association, always the strongest voice for those who have survived the triathlon of medical school and internship and private practice, had this to say about lobotomy:

> An emotional attitude of violent unreasoning opposition to the form of treatment [lobotomy] would be inexcusable. True it is a mutilating operation and it does result in certain defects in personality and behavior. However, much surgery is mutilating in the sense that some ordinary normal tissue is removed in order to achieve a beneficial result... No doctor can yet assert that this is or is not a truly worthwhile procedure. The ultimate decision must await the production of more scientific evidence.[2]

Dr. Watts wrote the chapters in *Psychosurgery* describing in detail not only how to perform a prefrontal lobotomy, but also the care of patients during the recovery period, advice for relatives, and the possible adverse effects. His detailed instructions and illustrations in this book made it possible for doctors in England, Japan, and elsewhere to perform this surgery. *Time* magazine reported that between September 14, 1936, the date of Freeman and Watts' first prefrontal lobotomy, and August 1949, there had been 10,706 lobotomies performed in the United States.[3] My father's lobotomy was one of those statistics, leaving him with losses in initiative, ambition, and creativity, not to mention the loss of his freedom and personality.

There were a few brave dissenting voices who spoke out against the American Medical Association's passive acquiescence to this mutilating operation. The following excerpt is from an editorial in the *Medical Record* entitled "The Lobotomy Delusion":

> Lobotomy for frontal lobe malignant tumor we can understand, but this is extended lobotomy, one is supposed to pluck from the brain a hidden sorrow... If the cutting of one set of frontal lobe association fibers is not sufficient, try cutting both sides, *i.e.*, analogously, if cutting off one leg of a paraplegic does not cure the individual, cut off both legs... To us the whole procedure...is medically wrong. Its

advocates overlook entirely the functions of the brain in the make up of the personality of the individual...

In the name of Madam Roland who cried aloud concerning the many crimes committed in the cause of liberty we would call the attention of those mutilating surgeons to the Hippocratic Oath.[4]

But Drs. Freeman and Watts were allowed to continue their crusade, even though more and more doctors saw what lobotomy left in its wake: men and women with not enough mental spark to dress themselves, let alone find a job; people who only remained alive because a nurse gave them nourishment through a tube. Many human beings died just because they didn't have enough fight left to keep from choking on their food. Bleeding was the most persistent and deadly complication from lobotomy.

The three months I worked as a student nurse at Toledo State Hospital I was assigned to a large ward with rows of cribs that held women who cried like infants every time anyone touched them. It was a warehouse for humans in diapers who moaned from painful contractures. My job was to feed one after the other, transfer them to gurneys, and wheel them down the hall to bathtubs. The wards were overcrowded. Patients in straitjackets were a common sight. Sedative packs (moist, cool sheets that were wrapped around the patient and then around the table) were common. Ward attendants could make life miserable; "pesty" patients could spend weeks in isolation. Patients were immersed for hours in water in continuous-flow tubs. As a student nurse, I, too, held the paddles during electroshock therapy and watched patients convulse into silence.

Even though I read his chart, I will never know if my father was diagnosed correctly as a schizophrenic or whether he simply was severely depressed over the passing of my baby sister and had no power to extricate himself from the psychiatric system once he became locked within their walls.

Days next to Grand Lake are treasures to be held in the hand, days to be measured for perfection against all others. Morning arrives calm, cool, fresh. Up even before the birds, I enjoy a mug of coffee by my favorite rock that faces Mount Baldy. A Douglas squirrel scolds me from further up the beach. He has far too much to say, but his big mouth is comic relief against shifting greens and grays. In October, Colorado air becomes thinner and colder and hoarfrost makes the ground look as if it were sprinkled with diamond dust.

The sound of water grows louder, small rapids ahead. I listen to the lake converse with itself, like two lovers reunited after a long absence. The northern inlet is made up of snow crystals that form chains of icy water that flow into Grand Lake. Indians, who first lived here, named the lake "Spirit Lake." Always water flows downhill, always head-over-heels, on its way to somewhere else.

Watching this river fill up the lake, year after year, renews my faith in the sense of goin-on-ness, progression. Grand Lake, with its bird calls and bombastic waves, its ruffles and riffles, the smell of wet clay, the magic marriage of visible and invisible, is a landscape that refreshes the eye, cleanses the heart, and recharges the spirit. Sunlight explodes through aspen leaves reminding me to look up. Faith is a pure element, like air and water and flame. For most of my life, poems and short stories and essays have been an outcry, a prayer, an offering.

Proust said that the real voyage of discovery was not seeing new landscapes but having new eyes. Georgia O'Keefe learned the artistic styles and devices that her teachers put forth but had not yet become an artist, because she still lacked her own vision. One day she went on a canoeing date with two men. The men were competitive and not behaving well. O'Keefe was miserable in their company. Suddenly, she noticed that, besides feeling privately awful, the day looked terrible as well. Its colors were dour and the shapes gloomy. She was struck by the realization that her feelings governed the way she saw the scene. It was a moment of transformation. The entire visual world, she realized, was dependent on the emotional world.

Toward the end of his life, Cezanne wondered whether his genius for painting might not have come from trouble with his eyes. Perhaps his whole life had been a mere accident of his body. Was it his myopia, the fact that he refused to wear glasses, or his diabetic condition that had caused retinal damage and cataracts, the clouding of the lens, that made him see the universe slightly askew but also uniquely beautiful?

Both my father and I were injured by medical treatments that were intended to help. My father's lobotomy caused irreversible brain damage. My vaccine-related illness caused systemic lupus. I am not against the administration of vaccines, but I only ask that patients be fully informed of the risks involved before they receive immunizations, including the fact that ethylmercury and formaldehyde are used in their preparation. The scandal of allowing a non-surgeon to perform thousands of lobotomies on helpless people locked up in mental institutions pales in comparison to the damage caused by injecting ethylmercury into our children. Meanwhile, the world witnesses the ever-growing epidemic of autistic and neurologically damaged children and all the infants who die for unknown reasons, forever labeled as "Sudden Infant Death Syndrome."

Shortly after receiving a hepatitis B vaccine booster shot, Lyla Rose Belkin died on September 16, 1998, at the age of five weeks. On February 18, 1999, in Atlanta, Georgia, her father, Michael Belkin, testified before the Advisory Committee on Immunization Practices Centers for Disease Control and Prevention that his daughter had been a lively, alert five-week-old baby when he held her in his arms the night before she died. She had never been ill before receiving the hepatitis B shot that afternoon. During her final feeding that night, she seemed agitated and feisty—and then fell asleep and didn't wake up. The only abnormality the coroner found was that the infant had a swollen brain. Lyla's pediatrician determined that "Sudden Infant Death Syndrome" was the cause of death, a catch-all diagnosis for unexplainable childhood mortality.

The grieving parents agonized over what symptoms they had missed or what they could have done differently, but the logical part of their brains always returned to the obvious medical event that had preceded their daughter's death.

"Could the hepatitis B vaccine that Lyla received that afternoon have killed her?" they asked physicians.

"The vaccine is perfectly safe," the doctors insisted.

However, when Belkin searched around on the Internet and Medline, he discovered disturbing evidence of adverse reactions to this vaccine. In the United States, the hepatitis B disease mainly infects intravenous drug users, homosexuals, prostitutes, and promiscuous heterosexuals. The disease is transmitted by blood. How could a newborn baby possibly get hepatitis B if the mother was screened and tested negative, as Lyla's mother had? Why were most U.S. babies inoculated at birth by their hospital or pediatrician with this vaccine?

The answer, Belkin discovered, was that an unrestrained health bureaucracy had decided that, since it couldn't get junkies, gays, prostitutes, and promiscuous heterosexuals to take the hepatitis B vaccine, they would mandate that all babies must be vaccinated at birth. Drug companies such as Merck, in their search for new markets, were instrumental in pushing government scientists to adopt an at-birth hepatitis B vaccination policy, although the vaccine had never been tested in newborns and no vaccines had ever been mandated at birth before.

Belkin's search for answers about his daughter's death led him to a hepatitis B vaccine workshop on October 26, 1999, at the National Academy of Sciences, Institute of Medicine entitled "Vaccine Safety Forum: Neonatal Deaths." The NAS was concerned enough about reports of hepatitis B vaccine-related infant deaths and adverse reactions to hold a special workshop on the subject. Doctors and scientists flew in from all over the U.S. and Europe to attend. There were basically four constituencies represented at this conference: 1. Serious scientists observing or presenting research studies; 2. Center for Disease Control pseudo-statisticians and FDA officials; 3. Merck and other corporate drug officials and 4. Parents of vaccine-related dead or severely injured children. Michael Belkin was amazed at what he heard.

One of the presentations was a study of "Animal Models of Newborn Response to Antigen Presentation," which showed that newborn immune systems were undeveloped and strikingly different than those of adults. A newborn's immune response to receiving shocks, such as being injected with a vaccine, was potentially unknown, since newborn T-cells, thymus-derived lymphocytes, have a radically different behavior than those of adults. Another presentation was "Strategies for Evaluating the Biologic Mechanisms of Hepatitis B Vaccine Reactions," in which vaccine researcher Dr. Bonnie Dunbar of Baylor University related numerous hepatitis B vaccine-related cases of nervous system damage in adults, such as multiple sclerosis, seizures, and blindness. On the more positive side, the FDA presented a seemingly reassuring study from its Vaccine Adverse Effects Reporting System (VAERS), which showed only nineteen neonatal deaths reported since 1991 related to hepatitis B vaccination.

But Michael Belkin knew that his daughter had died during their sample period and had not been counted. The New York City Coroner had called VAERS to report Lyla's hepatitis B vaccine-related infant death, and no one had ever returned his call.

"What kind of reporting system doesn't return the calls of the New York City Medical Examiner—and how many other reports were ignored?" Belkin wondered, as he sat in the room and listened in amazement as CDC officials and Merck's head of vaccine safety made disparaging comments about any possible risk from hepatitis B vaccination, despite the evidence just presented by impartial scientists. Their comments were scathingly dismissive of any possible risk from the vaccine.

Having studied statistics and econometrics at University of California, Berkeley, and having developed innovative methods of applying probability to financial and economic data in his consulting business, Michael Belkin was qualified to criticize the statistical legitimacy of the VAERS study, on which Merck and the CDC pseudo-scientist based their pro-vaccination stance. Obtaining raw data from the VAERS system, he found fifty-four reported SIDS cases after hepatitis B vaccination in just the eighteen months from January 1996 to May 1997, almost fifteen times as many deaths per year as their own flawed study had reported. There were seventeen thousand reports of adverse reactions to hepatitis B vaccine in the 1996-1997 raw data. Clearly, something was fishy about VAERS.

Belkin came away from that NAS workshop with the distinct impression that Merck and the CDC didn't really want to know how many babies were being killed or injured by the hepatitis B vaccination. "This is a bureaucratic vaccination program that is on auto-pilot flying into a mountain," Belkin said.

The Center for Disease Control bureaucrats had a vested interest in the status quo. If there had been seventeen thousand reports of a dangerous disease discovered during an eighteen-month period, the CDC would have been all over the case. But when there were seventeen thousand reports of adverse reactions to a vaccine the CDC advocated for "public health," the CDC dismissed it as a coincidence. Merck made fifty dollars per shot from the three-shot series and had sales of upwards of eight hundred million dollars per year from vaccines.

Belkin was convinced that the hepatitis B vaccine had not been administered for the well-being of his child. Rather, it had been delivered by the long arm of an incompetent and mindless bureaucracy, in the name of stamping out a disease most babies couldn't possibly get. The Drug Company/CDC/FDA alliance had pulled the wool over the medical profession's eyes with the hepatitis B vaccine. The American Academy of Pediatrics had bought the alliance's sales pitch and had recommended that all infants get this vaccine at birth. Babies were inflicted with a shock to their immune systems from a vaccine against a nonexistent risk of contracting hepatitis B. Nothing would bring his daughter, Lyla, back, but Michael Belkin vowed to speak out in the hope that other needless deaths and injuries might be prevented.

⌒ ⌒

In his article entitled "Deadly Immunity: Robert F. Kennedy Jr. investigates our government cover-up of a mercury/autism scandal," the author states that after analyzing the medical records of one hundred thousand children, CDC epidemiologist Tom Verstraeten concluded that thimerosal appeared to be responsible for the epidemic of autism and other neurological disorders among children. Dr. Verstraeten's study was suppressed by the CDC and the FDA out of fear of lawsuits from parents of injured children. When his study was finally published in 2003, he was employed by GlaxoSmithKline and had reworked the data from his research to hide the causative link between thimerosal and autism.[5]

By 1991, the estimated number of autistic children had increased fifteenfold, from one in every twenty-five hundred children, to one in 166 children. In 2007, the ratio is one child out of 150 are suffering from autism or other neurological and cognitive disabilities. In the United States alone, more than five hundred thousand children suffer from autism. Thimerosal was first used as a preservative in baby vaccines in 1931; the first diagnosed cases of autism appeared in 1943. By 1999, our government mandated that children should receive twenty-two immunizations by the time they reached first grade. No one bothered to add up how much ethylmercury was being injected into our children if they received the recommended inoculations. At two months of age, infants routinely received three inoculations containing a total of 62.5 micrograms of ethylmercury—a level ninety-nine times greater than the EPA's limit for daily exposure to methylmercury, a related neurotoxin. The only reason pharmaceutical companies add thimerosal to vaccines is so that they can get multiple doses out of the bottle. Our children are being harmed because the pharmaceutical companies want to increase the profits of their shareholders. We are in a moral crisis in America. If, as the evidence provided in Kennedy's article suggests, our public-health authorities have knowingly allowed the pharmaceutical industry to poison our children, we will see the repercussions for decades to come.

The Coalition for Mercury-free Drugs (CoMed), filed a lawsuit in August 2006 to compel the Food and Drug Administration (FDA) to provide proof of the safety and efficacy of mercury used in the manufacture of drugs as diverse as eye ointments, ear solutions, nasal sprays, biologics, and perhaps most importantly, in flu vaccines being administered to millions of pregnant women, children, and the elderly. Mercury, second only to plutonium in toxicity to humans, has been implicated in a long list of chronic disorders including Alzheimer's disease, asthma, attention-deficit disorder, autism, diabetes, and multiple sclerosis, among others. The FDA has acknowledged that mercury could easily be eliminated from the preparation of drugs. In a 1999 internal e-mail obtained under a Freedom of Information Act (FOIA) request, an FDA official admitted that the agency's failure to evaluate the cumulative amount of mercury in medicine, "will raise questions about FDA being 'asleep at the switch' for decades by allowing a potentially hazardous compound to remain…and not forcing manufacturers to exclude it from new products…"[6]

I fling open the windows, light candles, and buy roses for my table. I bury the memory of medical treatments and surgery and insomnia under the rich aroma of chopped onions and broccoli and red peppers as they simmer on the stove. *Be patient. Love is a laughing song that is written the more you sing.* The copper teapot gurgles on the stove. Resting firmly on the soles of my feet, there's nowhere I need to be except here in my kitchen waiting for the water to boil. Impatience is the illness. No need to hurry, no need to grasp. Sun streams in through the kitchen window. A meadowlark sings. My hand rummages through packets of tea: cinnamon, apple spice, rosehips, chamomile. I feel the cold metal teapot handle in the palm of my hand. I feel the cold faucet, hear the sound of water as it splashes against metal, feel heat as it curls up around the pot. No war, no struggle for control, no wanting to be someone or someplace else. Water mixes with tea. Cinnamon apple spice steeping. Each moment received is a gift. Sufficient. The touch of warm tea on my thirsty tongue is healing.

Sometimes it sings hymns, often the blues, but always the body hums along. Even a tuned and polished piano cannot soar with joy if the musician chooses grief. Scalpels can cut out tumors but cannot mend the damage done when a person's creativity is crushed. Chemicals cannot ease the pain of a suffering soul. Health is a matter of the heart, of what I digest or eliminate in my life, of being able to hear and see, to be able to stand on my own, the ability to handle crises. Healing is a process, a journey toward balance, connectedness, meaning, and wholeness, rather than an outcome.

Those treating the chronically ill enter a distant country with few markers, like those unexplored portions of maps in ancient times that carried the warning, "From here on, dragons!" By definition, a chronic illness, like lupus, cannot be cured. Quest for a cure is a dangerous myth that serves both patient and doctor poorly. The goal should be to reduce the frequency and severity of exacerbations in the course of chronic illness. My goal is to maintain independence, to find purpose and joy in each day.

Words hold the power to wound or heal. My father was labeled as "crazy." My mother and I were labeled as "invalid." *In-valid. Not worthy.* I, among others in the disabled community, prefer "disabled," or even better, "person with a disability," since it emphasizes the person behind the condition. It is always the person, the story, discovering why any of us have been given the gift of life and why we fight so hard to keep on going. What constitutes salvation? Something bestowed by an unseen God or something that each of us must find for himself or herself?

Body language is music I get under my fingers, synapses in the brain, body as vessel for sound and feeling. Voice is the body given away in the world. Voice is making love. Speech is intimate, a sacred art, making the inner and outer world one. Voice is re-owning my body, and the joy I receive from writing every day is the physical "ah-ha" of the soul. *Cultivate silence. Become the rest between two notes that are always in discord. Pay more attention to the current than the rocks in the river. Longing is your teacher. Keep feeding your desires. Breath is the cycle of rest, the way of paying attention to the universe. Say yes instead of no.*

⌒ ⌒

The year of Jubilee in the Bible was when Moses led the Jews into their promised land. Jubilee is the name of the cabin I build in Grand Lake, Colorado, a small town high up in the Rocky Mountains. The first step is finding a builder whom I can trust, a mountain man who carries on a love affair with his sixteen-ounce hammer and twelve-penny nails, an artist who uses wood to build something of permanence, like a classic book that has earned its place high on the shelf. He is an expert at shoveling dirt, pouring forms for the footer, pounding wooden stakes into earth. Wielding hammer and nail and saw, he squares and levels earth, as if we have power. There is no turning back once ground is broken.

When not even one wall has been raised, I dream of a plume of smoke rising from the chimney, Vivaldi rolling down hallways. There will be two decks and nooks and crannies, lots of windows looking out to lodgepole pines, and down the driveway, Grand Lake. So many decisions to make—square footage, fireplace, countertop, carpet—but all things are possible, like Thoreau, who found the universe in the length and breadth and depth of his pond. Peace of mind flows in as I sit by the lake, where trees reflect their true selves with no masks, no arrogance. Building a house, like writing, is faith that joints will come close enough for putty to cover, that the wood will swell and close any gaps in design. Wind whistles and wails above the trees like an angry mountain god, and in early twilight, gossamer nymphs and fairies flutter through gauzy, gray-green tree moss. Magic is still here.

When finished, my home is more beautiful than I had ever dreamed possible, a hand-crafted house, so loving in each detail. Reflected light from the snow off the Rockies holds a clarity and beauty not seen anywhere else. Winter sun spews gold across the rug. I sit on the porch at Jubilee and enjoy a gorgeous autumn afternoon. Water from the river sings over rocks as it flows into Grand Lake, sparkling through lodgepole pines.

"You're a little closer to Heaven when you're in Grand Lake," the plaque hanging on my wall says. Freedom is not about having nothing left to lose but nothing left to be. Watching the lake is better than any sermon from a pulpit, as it demonstrates the healing power of nature. Set free in the middle of my life, sun is warm on my back. Hawks do their call-and-response routine: "Amen. Amen." I'm home.

I think about my father while I pull weeds in my yard. There is silence. No birds sing, no woodpeckers, no chipmunks, or crickets. Heat waves shimmer before me. The rocks and trees look as if I were looking through a century-old windowpane, wavy imperfections running through glass. I wonder if my father realized what had happened to him, whether the knowledge had come to him all at once or built slowly over time.

Here among the anthills and worm dungeons and dandelions, I close my eyes and a powerful image rises up. I am arguing with God, scolding Him for being cruel and indifferent, when His thundering voice exclaims, "Isn't faith the treasure hidden in the field, the pearl of great price? Didn't I give you a father to teach you love? And didn't he do his best to provide for you? Didn't he make you laugh and fill you with joy and excitement and renew your own ragged sense of wonder?"

"Yes, but why did you take him away from me?" I ask.

"Because wisdom and strength and love are born out of suffering. Is that so difficult to understand? Must everything be perfect to satisfy you?" Embarrassed by my selfishness and ignorance, I silently continue weeding.

"Watch," God says, and suddenly it is Judgment Day, and all the men and women in mental institutions and hospitals, with their waxen faces and staggering gaits and silenced voices, sweep through unlocked gates into the sun. In a vast green field, they join hands in an ecstatic, golden dance. One by one, they jump and soar, whirling and rolling like ballet dancers, while their daughters and mothers and fathers form a circle around them, clapping. The air vibrates with cheers and whistles. When Father is exhausted, he walks slowly but erectly toward me with outstretched hands.

"I've never left you, Connie. Marguerite and your mother haven't either," Father says. "Don't you see?" When I open my eyes, they are burning with tears.

"Yes, I see," I say, as I pull a thistle from my bed of petunias.

NOTES

1. Freeman, Walter and James W. Watts. *Psychosurgery: Intelligence, Emotion and Social Behavior.* (Springfield, IL: Charles C. Thomas, 1942), 27.
2. "Frontal Lobotomy," *Journal of the American Medical Association* 117 (16 August 1941): 534-35.
3. *Time*, 23 December 1946, 67.
4. "The Lobotomy Delusion," *Medical Record* (15 May 1940): 335.
5. Kennedy, Robert F. Jr.. "Deadly Immunity: Robert F. Kennedy Jr. investigates the government cover-up of a mercury/autism scandal," *Rolling Stone Magazine*, 2005, 977-88.
6. Put Children First. 29 June 1999. www.putchildrenfirst.org/media/1.6.pdf.

Bibliography

Books:

Coulter, Harris L. *Vaccination, Social Science, and Criminality: The Medical Assault on the American Brain.* Berkeley, CA: North Atlantic Books, 1990.

————., and Barbara Loe Fisher. *A Shot In The Dark.* Garden City Park, NY: Avery Publishing Group, Inc., 1991.

Freeman, Walter, and James W. Watts. *Psychosurgery: Intelligence, Emotion and Social Behavior.* Springfield, IL: Charles C. Thomas, 1942.

Gardner, W. H., and N. H. MacKenzie, eds. *The Poems of Gerard Manley Hopkins.* New York: Oxford University Press, 1967.

James, Walene. *Immunization: The Reality Behind the Myth.* South Hadley, MA: Bergin & Garvey Publishers, Inc., 1988.

Miller, Neil Z. *Immunization: Theory vs. Reality.* Santa Fe: New Atlantean Press, 1996.

————. *Vaccines: Are They Really Safe and Effective?: A Parent's Guide To Childhood Shots.* Santa Fe: New Atlantean Press, 1992.

Murphy, Jamie. *What Every Parent Should Know About Childhood Immunization.* Boston: Earth Healing Products, 1993.

Neustaedter, Randall. *The Vaccine Guide: Making An Informed Choice.* Berkeley: North Atlantic Books, Homeopathic Educational Services, 1996.

Scheibner, Viera. *Vaccination: 100 Years of Orthodox Research Shows that Vaccines Represent an Assault on the Immune System.* Victoria: Australian Print Group, 1993.

Stratton, Kathleen R. Cynthia J. How, and Richard B. Johnson, Jr., eds. *Adverse Events Associated With Childhood Vaccines: Evidence Bearing On Causality.* Washington, DC: National Academy Press, 1994.

Valenstein, Elliot S. *Great and Desperate Cures: The Rise and Decline of Psychosurgery and Other Radical Treatments for Mental Illness.* New York: Basic Books, Inc., 1986.

ARTICLES:

Allen, M. B., et al. "Pulmonary and cutaneous vasculitis following hepatitis B vaccination." *Thorax* 48, no. 5 (May 1993): 580-1.

Alter, M. J., S. C. Hadler, H. S. Margolis, J. Alexander, et al. "The changing epidemiology of hepatitis B in the United States." *Journal of the American Medical Association* 263, no. 9 (2 March 1990): 1218-22.

Ballinger, A. B., M. L. Clark. "Severe acute hepatitis B infection after vaccination." *Lancet* 344 (8932): 1292-3.

Belkin, Michael. Transcript, testimony before the Advisory Committee on Immunization Practices Centers for Disease Control and Prevention, Atlanta, GA, February 18, 1999.

Biasi, D. "Rheumatological Manifestations Following Hepatitis B Vaccination. A Report of 2 Clinical Cases." [English abstract.] *Recenti Progressi Medicina* 85, no. 9 (September 1985): 438-40.

Birley, H. D. "Hepatitis B and Reactive Arthritis." [Letter.] *British Medical Journal* 309, no. 6967 (3 December 1994): 1514.

Blair, A., P. Stewart, M. O'Berg, et al. "Mortality among industrial workers exposed to formaldehyde." *Journal of the National Cancer* Institute 76, no. 6 (1986): 1071-84.

————., R. Saracci, P. A. Stewart, et al. "Epidemiologic evidence on the relationship between formaldehyde exposure and cancer." *Scandinavian Journal of Work, Environment and Health* 16, no. 6 (1990): 381-393.

Caulfield, M. "Hepatitis B: A Disease Needing a Vaccine or a Vaccine Needing a Disease?" *Clinical Pediatrics (Philadelphia)* 32, no. 7 (1993): 443-4.

Centers for Disease Control. "Hepatitis B virus: a comprehensive strategy for eliminating transmission in the United States through universal childhood vaccination. Recommendations of the Immunization Practices Advisory Committee (ACIP)." *Morbidity and Mortality Weekly Report)* 41, no. SS-6 (1992, b): 1-13.

Clement International Corporation. "Toxicological profile for mercury." *U.S. Department of Health and Human Services, Public Health Service, Agency for Toxic Substances and Disease Registry.* Washington, DC, 1992.

Dhaffin, D., B. Dinman, J. Miller, et al. "An evaluation of the effects of chronic mercury exposure on EMG and psychomotor functions." *U.S. Department of Health and Human Services, National Institute of Occupational Safety and Health.* Document no. HSM-099-71-62, Washington, DC, 1973.

"FDA Accused of Not Investigating Adverse Reactions to Vaccines." *U.S. Medicine* (November 1992): 32.

Fenichel, G.M. "Neurological complications of immunization." *Annals of Neurology* 12 (1982):119-28.

Freed, G. L., W. C. Bordley, S. J. Clark, and T. R. Konrad. "Reactions of pediatricians to a new Centers for Disease Control recommendation for universal immunization of infants with hepatitis B vaccine." *Pediatrics* 91 (1993):699-702.

Fulginiti, V. A. "Controversies in current immunization policies and practices." *Current Problems in Pediatrics* 6 (1976):6-16.

Goffin, E., Y. Horsmans, C. Cornu, et al. "Acute hepatitis B infection after vaccination." [Letter.] *Lancet* 345 (1995):263.

Gross, K., C. Combe, K. Kruger, and M. Schattenkirchner. "Arthritis after hepatitis vaccination: report of 3 cases." *Scandinavian Journal Rheumatology* 24 (1995):50-52.

Hachulla, E., E. Houvenagel, A. Mingui, G. Vincent, and A. Laine. A. "Reactive arthritis after hepatitis B vaccination." *Journal of Rheumatology* 17 (1990): 1250-51.

Hadler, S. C., D. P. Francis, J. E. Maynard, et al. "Long-term immunogenicity and efficacy of hepatitis B vaccine in homosexual men." *New England Journal of Medicine* 315 (1986):209-14.

Hall, A. J. "Hepatitis B vaccination: protection for how long and against what? Booster injections are not indicated." *British Medical Journal* 307 (1993):276-77.

Hall, C. B., and N. A. Halsey. "Control of hepatitis B: to be or not to be?" *Pediatrics* 90 (1992): 274-77.

Hayes, R. B., J. W. Raatgever, A. de Bruyn, and M. Gerin. "Cancer of the nasal cavity and paranasal sinuses, and formaldehyde exposure." *International Journal of Cancer* 37, no. 4 (1986):487-92.

"Hepatitis B Vaccines—To Switch Or Not To Switch." *Journal of the American Medical Association* 257 (1987):2634-36.

Herroelen, L., J. DeKeyser, and G. Ebinger. "Central-nervous-system demyelination after immunization with recombinant hepatitis B vaccine." *Lancet* 338 (1991):1174-75.

Hirszel, P., J. H. Michaelson, K. Dodge, et al. "Mercury-induced autoimmune glomerulonephritis in inbred rats—part II. Immunohistopathology, histopathology and effects of prostaglandin administration." *Survey Synth Pathological Research* 4 (1985):412-22.

Jawad, A. S., and D. G. Scott. "Immunization triggering rheumatoid arthritis?" *Annals of Rheumatic Disease* 48 (1989):174.

Kennedy, Robert F. Jr. "Deadly Immunity: Robert F. Kenndy Jr. investigates the government cover-up of a mercury/autism scandal." *Rolling Stone Magazine* 977/988.

Lear, J. T., et al. "Anaphylaxis After Hepatitis B Vaccine." [Letter.] *Lancet* 345, no 8959 (13 May 1995): 1249.

Lilic, D., and S. K. Ghosh. "Liver dysfunction and DNA antibodies after hepatitis B vaccination." *Lancet* 344 (1994): 1292-93.

Mamoux, V. "Lupus E. Disseminatus and Vaccination Against Hepatitis B Virus." [Letter.] *Archives Pediatrics* 1, no. 3 (1994): 307-8.

Martinez, E., and P. Domingo. "Evan's syndrome triggered by recombinant hepatitis B vaccine." *Clinical Infectious Diseases* 15 (1992):1051.

McEwen, M. "Should there be universal childhood vaccination against hepatitis B?" *Pediatric Nursing* 19 (1993):447-52.

McIntyre., P. J., "Acute Hepatitis B Infection After Vaccination." [Letter.] *Lancet* 345, no. 8944 (28 January 1995): 261-63.

"Mds Resist Hepatitis B Vaccine Mandate for Infants as Safety Questions Surface About Immunizations." *Health Facts: Center for Medical Consumers* (August 1993): 1.

Mendelsohn, R. "The truth about immunizations." *The People's Doctor* (April 1978): 1.

Morris, J. A., and H. Butler. "Nature and frequency of adverse reaction following hepatitis B vaccine injection in children in New Zealand, 1985-1988." Submitted to the Vaccine Safety Committee, Institute of Medicine, Washington, DC, 4 May 1992.

Moskowitz, R. "The case against immunizations: Directions for future research." *Journal of the American Institute of Homeopathy* 78 (1985): 101-4.

———. "Immunizations: The other side." *Mothering* 31 (1984):32-38.

———. "Vaccination: A sacrament of modern medicine." *Journal of the American Institute of Homeopathy* 84 (1991): 96-105.

Nadler, J. P. "Multiple Sclerosis and Hepatitis B Vaccine." [Letter.] Clinical Infectious Diseases, 5 (17 November 1993): 928-29.

Poullin, P., and B. Gabriel. "Thrombocytopenic purpura after recombinant hepatitis B vaccine." *Lancet* 344 (1994): 1293.

Ribera, E. F., and A. J. Dutka. "Polyneuropathy associated with administration of hepatitis B vaccine." *New England Journal of Medicine* 309 (1983):614-15.

Rietshcel, R. L., and R. M. Adams. "Reactions to thimerosol in hepatitis B vaccines." *Dermatologic Clinics* 8 (1990):161-64.

Scheibner, Viera. "The Vaccination Debate." *Natural Health* (August/September 1991).

Shaw, F. E., D. J. Graham, H. A. Guess, J. B. Milstien, et al. "Postmarketing surveillance for neurologic adverse events reported after hepatitis B vaccination: Experience of the first three years." *American Journal of Epidemiology* 127 (1988):337-52.

Simpson, N., L. Simon, and R. Randall. "Parental refusal to have children immunized: extent and reasons." *British Medical Journal* 310 (1995):227.

Street, A. C., T. Z. Weddle, W. R. Thomann, E. W. Lundbert, et al. "Persistence of antibody in healthcare workers vaccinated against hepatitis B." *Infection Control and Hospital Epidemiology* 11 (1990):525-30.

Tosti, A., M. Melino, and F. Bardazzi. "Systemic reactions due to thimerosal." *Contact Dermatitis* 15 (1986):187-88.

Trevisani, F., G. C. Gattinara, P. Caraceni, M. Bernardi, et al. "Transverse myelitis following hepatitis B vaccination." *Journal of Hepatology* 19 (1993):317-18.

Tudela, P., et al. "Systemic Lupus and Vaccination Against Hepatitis B." [Letter.] *Nephron* 62, no. 2 (1992): 236.

"Vaccines and Victims." *Insight on the News* (5 April 1992): 6.

Vautier, G., and J. E. Carty. "Acute sero-positive rheumatoid arthritis occurring after hepatitis vaccination." *British Journal of Rheumatology* 33 (1994): 991.

ORGANIZATIONS:

The National Vaccine Information Center (NVIC)
512 W. Maple Avenue
Vienna, VA 22180
1-800-909-SHOT

The Coalition for Mercury-free Drugs (CoMeD)
(http://www.mercury-freedrugs.org)

Advocates for Children's Health Affected by Mercury Poisoning (A-CHAMP)
(http://www.a-champ.org)